You are
what you eat

This book has been published to accompany a series of
eight radio programmes 'You are what you Eat'.
First broadcast on Mondays from March 29th 1976
on Radio 3 Medium Wave at 6.30 p.m.

Repeated in 1977.

The series produced by Michael Totton.

Published to accompany a series of
programmes prepared in consultation with
the BBC Further Education Advisory Council.

© the Author
First published 1976
Published by the British Broadcasting Corporation
35 Marylebone High Street, London W1M 4AA
ISBN 0 563 10994 7
Printed in England by John Blackburn Limited.
This book is printed in Monophoto 10/11pt Ehrhardt.

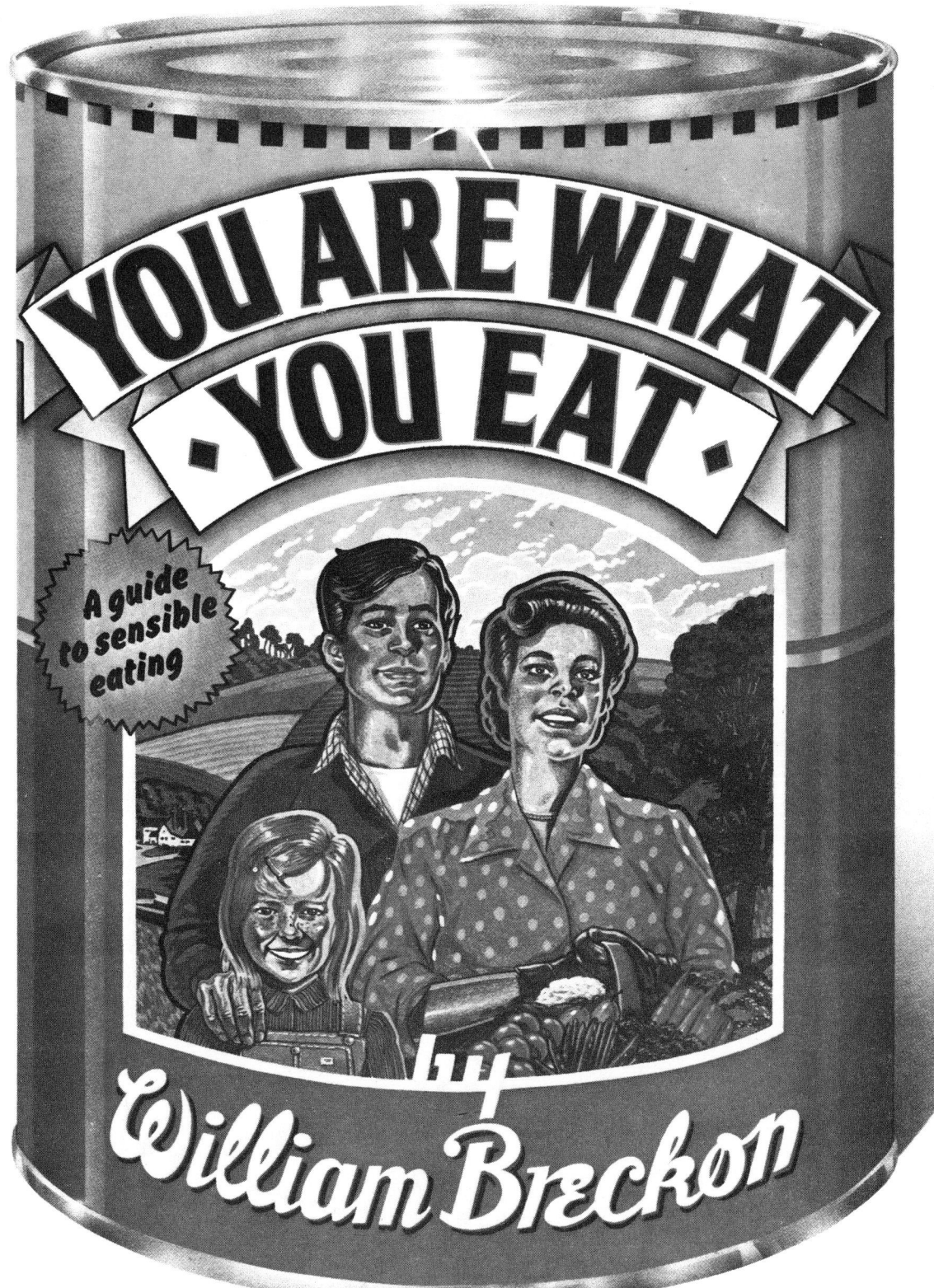

YOU ARE WHAT
·YOU EAT·

A guide to sensible eating

by

William Breckon

BRITISH BROADCASTING CORPORATION

Contents

1 Eating Habits

Alas, what various tastes in food
Divide the human brotherhood!
Birds in their little nests agree
With Chinamen but not with me.
Colonials like their oysters hot,
Their omelettes heavy – I do not.
The French are fond of slugs and frogs
The Siamese eat puppy dogs . . .

Hilaire Belloc' 'On Food'.

What will not luxury taste? Earth, sea and air
Are daily ransacked for the bill of fare.
Blood stuffed in skins is British Christian's food
And France robs marshes of the croaking brood.

John Gay, 'Trivia'.

The food we eat is governed not so much by what nutrients are readily available but more by habit, history, custom and taboo. Our earliest forebears doubtless grabbed at anything – root, berry or leaf, fish, flesh or fowl – which, by experience, they learned was both nutritious and non-poisonous. Modern man, however, is a fussy eater, at least in the sense that ethnic groups or communities have tended to confine themselves to diets based on only a few species of cereals, root crops, vegetables and fruits and the products of a very limited number of animals.

Even so it is still very much true that one man's meat in one part of the world is the poison of his brother in another.

Such differences bedevil the work of any nutritionist who seeks to introduce a rational (to his mind), well-balanced diet to a community where there is nutritional deprivation. Some of the recent famines in India have had as their basic cause the failure of the rice crop – the traditional staple food. But attempts by famine relief workers to overcome the problem by substituting wheat for rice have often foundered on dislike of so novel a food, and deep ingrained suspicion of it.

As Magnus Pyke has written in *Food and Society*: 'The fact remains that men and women living in the societies which make up the human population do not ingest nutrients, they consume foods. More than this, they eat meals. Although to the single-minded chemist or physiologist, this aspect of human behaviour may appear to be irrelevant or even frivolous, it is nevertheless a deeply ingrained part of the human situation which exerts a very direct and profound effect on nutritional status and health.'

Dr Pyke adds: 'In few areas of human behaviour do the early conditioning of customary use and inbred tradition exert so subtle an effect on the mind, not only of the people being studied, but of the scientific investigator as well. Few Englishwomen trained to use all their intellectual facilities at Oxford University, stop to question the truth of what they assert with such authority to their husbands and children, that a *hot* breakfast of porridge, bacon and eggs is essential for proper nutrition, regardless of the evidence of the millions outside England who subsist without these items in the morning.' Ludwig Feuerbach's assertion that we are what we eat may not be strictly true in the sense that no matter what exotic foods we ingest they are quickly broken

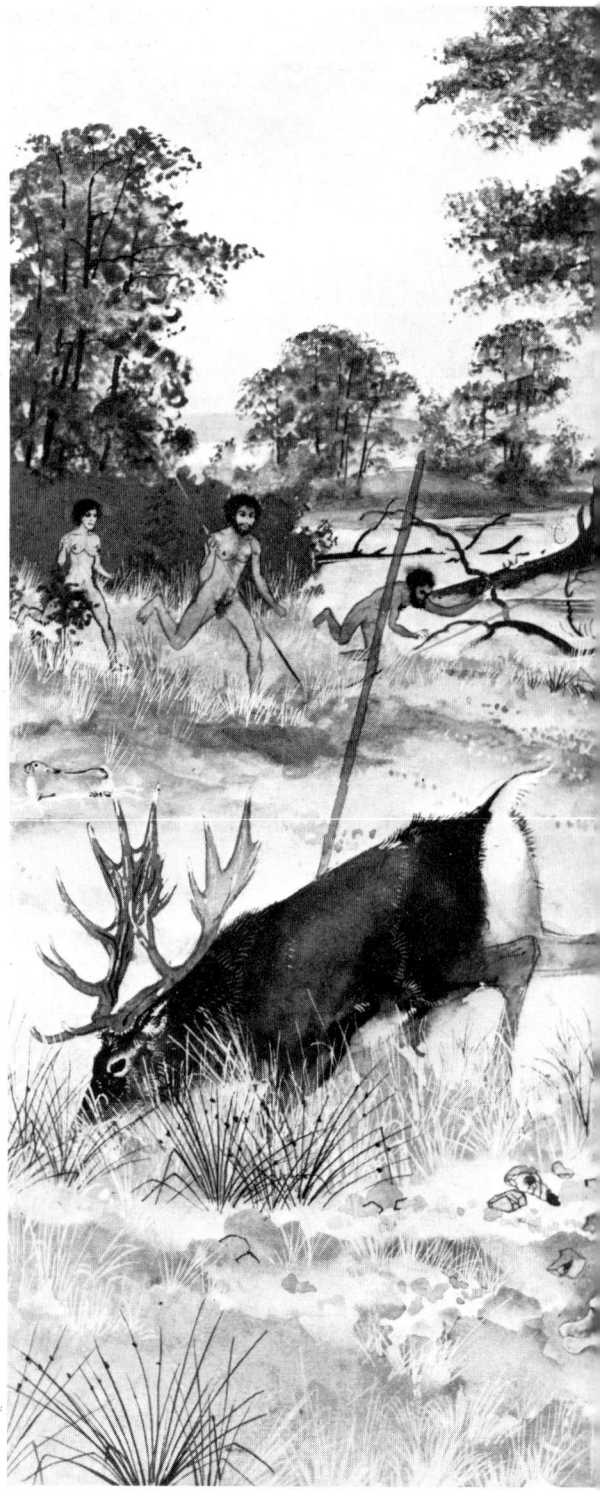

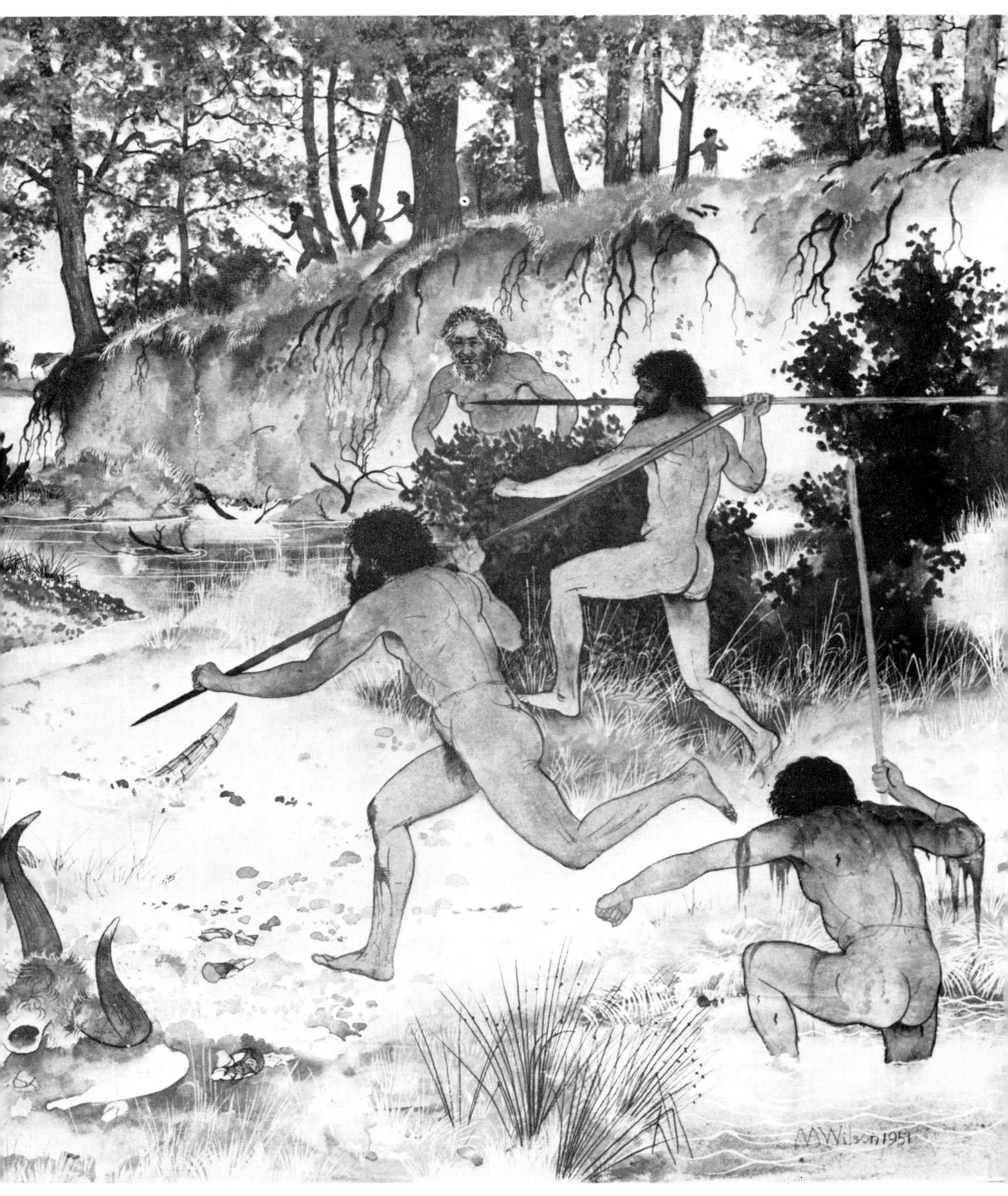

Hunting scene: Old Stone Age.

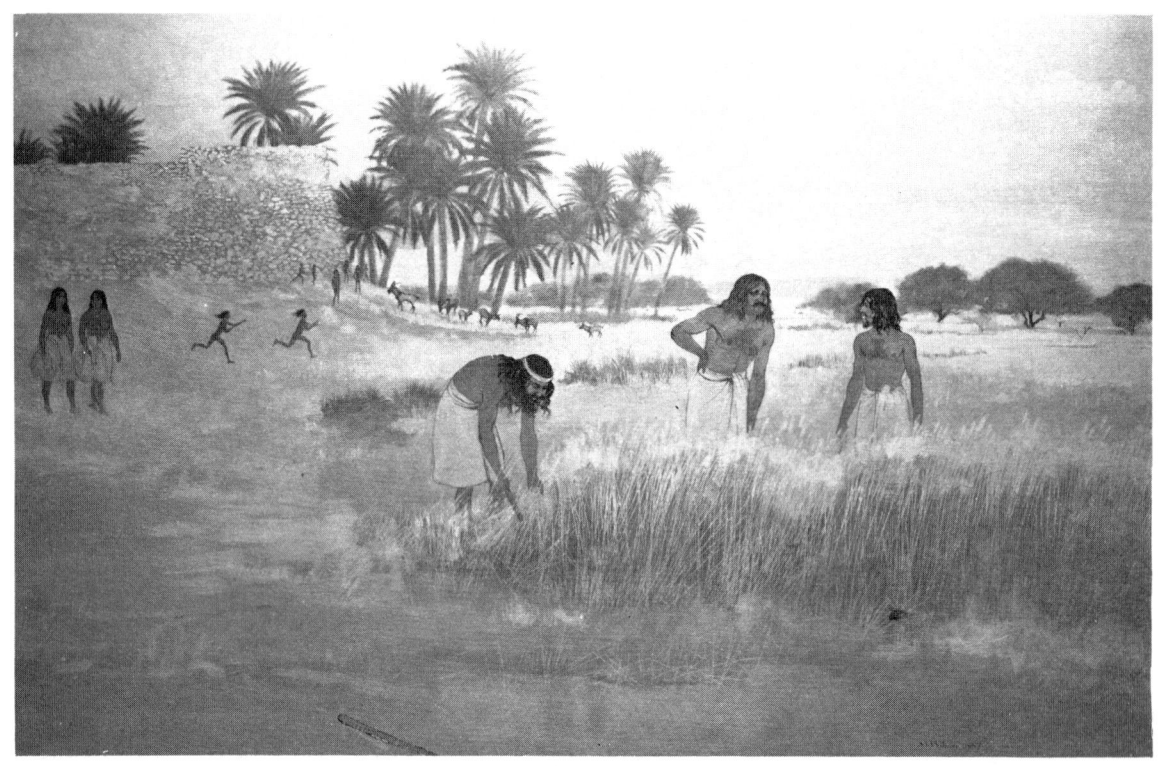

The Neolithic Revolution: settled agriculture.

down into the same basic chemical nutrients. But major differences in dietary habits in general can have a considerable effect on life-styles. (And vice-versa, for what we are, as far as ethnic group and social status is concerned, largely influences what we eat.)

One cardinal example of this is to be found in a classic study carried out by Dr J. G. Orr (later Lord Boyd Orr) and Dr J. L. Gilks on the Kikuyu and Masai peoples in Africa. At the time of the survey (it was published in 1931) the Kikuyu were a settled agricultural race with a mainly vegetarian diet while the Masai were pastoral and as well as eating vegetables and cereals, ate the meat of, and drank the milk from, their cattle. They also, from time to time, drank blood which they drew from live beasts without harming them.

The differences between these two neighbouring races was striking: the Masai were on average five inches taller, 23 lbs heavier and had a 50 per cent greater muscular strength then the Kikuyu. The latter, whose diet was mainly carbohydrate, were found to be much more prone

to disease, subject to lethargy and lacking in stamina. Some 63 per cent of the Kikuyu boys had bone deformities, compared with 12 per cent of the Masai boys; 40 per cent had decayed teeth compared with just eight per cent among the Masai; 48 per cent of the Kikuyu boys suffered from anaemia, while only 12 per cent of the Masai boys did so.

Of course, not all these differences can be laid at diet's door, but Drs Orr and Gilks were convinced that the Kikuyu's inferiorities were due in very large measure to what they ate.

Similar pronounced differences were found in India earlier in the century by Sir Robert McCarrison. He wrote: 'Nothing could be more striking than the contrast between the manly, stalwart and resolute races of the North – the Pathans, Baluchis, Sikhs, Punjabis, Rajputs and Maharattas – and the poorly-developed, toneless and supine people of the East and South; Bengalis, Madrassis, Kanarese and Travancorians.'

McCarrison tested various Indian diets on groups of young rats. Some, for example, were

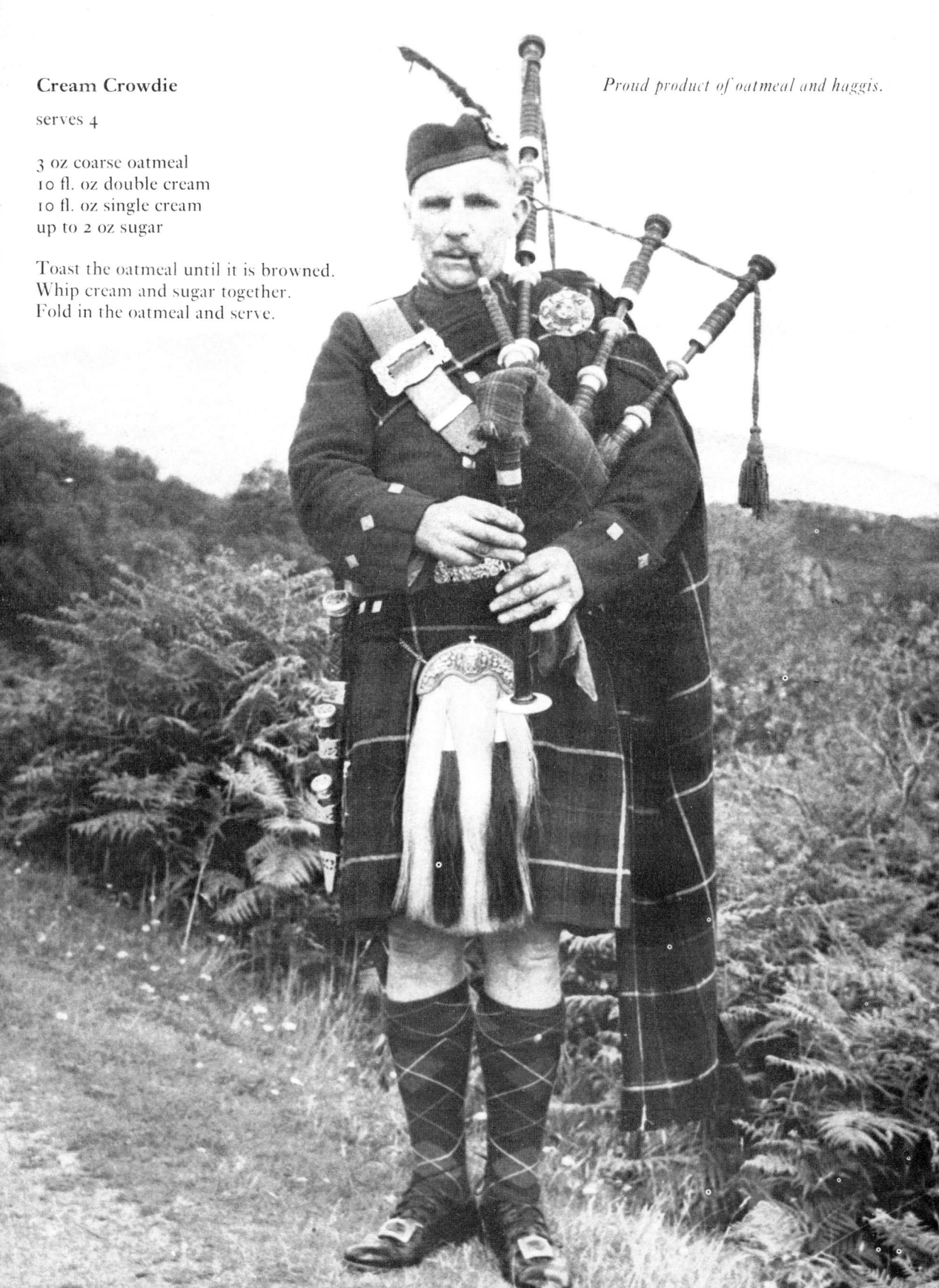

Cream Crowdie

Proud product of oatmeal and haggis.

serves 4

3 oz coarse oatmeal
10 fl. oz double cream
10 fl. oz single cream
up to 2 oz sugar

Toast the oatmeal until it is browned.
Whip cream and sugar together.
Fold in the oatmeal and serve.

Yorkshire Pudding

serves 6

4 oz plain flour
pinch salt
1 egg
10 fl. oz milk (or milk and water)

Mix flour and salt. Make a well in it and put in the
egg and a little milk. Working from the middle,
stir into a batter, gradually adding rest of milk.

Have the beef roasting on a rack *above* the pan,
at 425°F (Gas mark 7). Allow 15 min. per pound
for rare beef.

40 minutes before the end of roasting, pour
batter into the pan. It will rise up at the sides, and
the juices will collect in the middle.

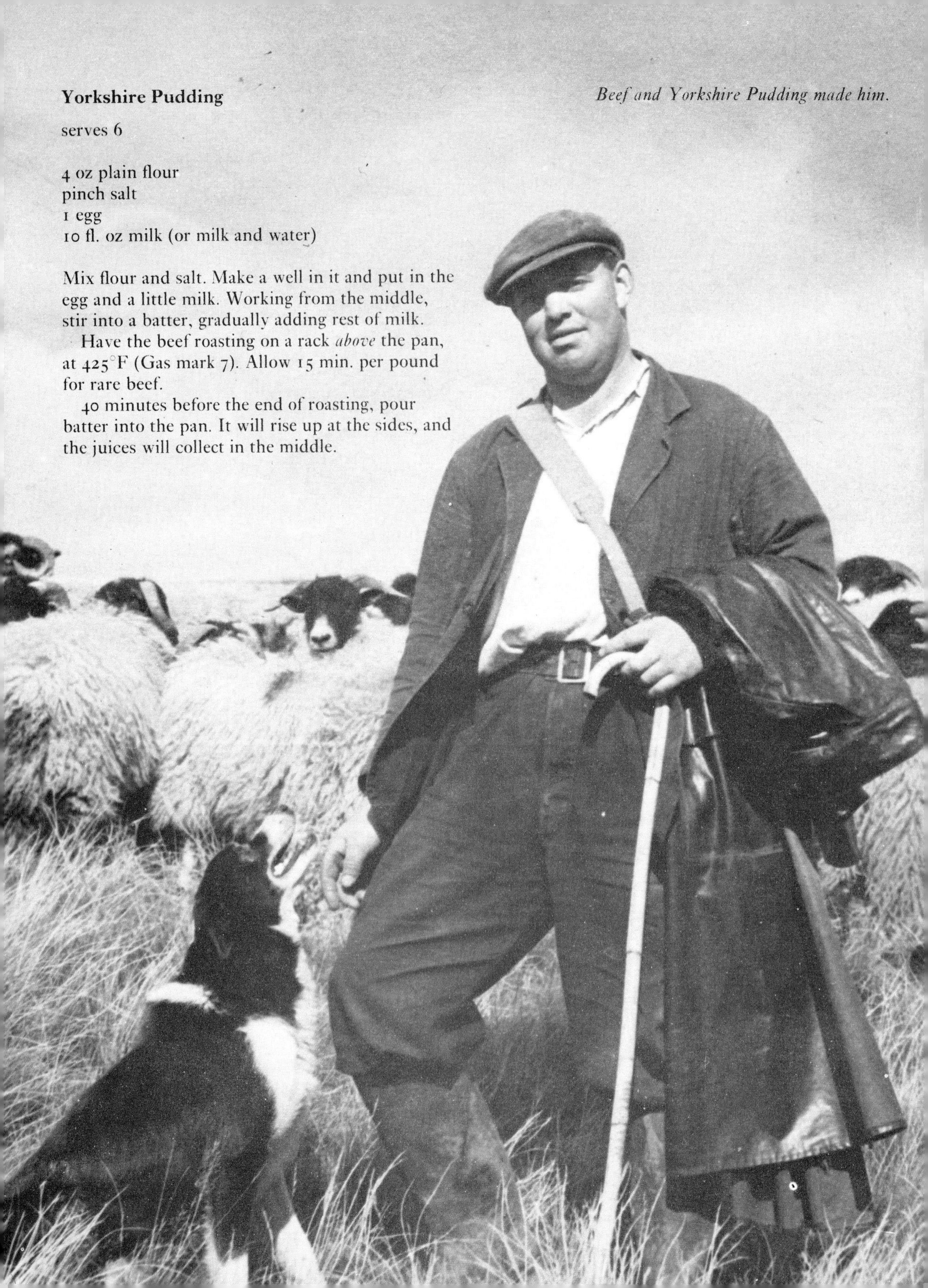

Beef and Yorkshire Pudding made him.

given a standard Sikh diet: unleavened bread made from freshly-ground whole wheat, milk, butter, curds, ghee (clarified butter), legumes and various vegetables. They had meat just once a week. Other rats were fed the standard Madrassi diet of polished rice and legumes, various condiments and vegetable oil, far less ghee, coffee with sugar and a little milk, and coconut.

By the end of the trial the 'Sikh' rats weighed an average of 235 grams while the 'Madrassis' weighed only 155 grams.

Regarding the differences in physique and temperament between the human races in India, Sir Robert concluded: 'Inherited factors, climate, customs, caste, religion and endemic diseases no doubt contribute their share to the production of this result; but food is the paramount factor concerned.'

Old wives' tales

It is tempting, but dangerous, to suggest that other regional and national differences may be due to diet. What true Scotsman would deny his fierce patriotism and physical strength derive from daily porridge and well-blooded haggis! Does not the Yorkshireman's bluffness and doggedness come from the consumption of a plethora of puddings – blood, black and batter?

Unfortunately a close scientific examination reveals no basis for such claims. There is a little regional variation in the total consumption of the basic nutrients – proteins, carbohydrates, fats, vitamins and minerals – but by no means enough to explain the varying characteristics. Scotsmen and Yorkshiremen are what they are for many different inherited, climatic and cultural reasons, not for what they eat. Only when there are gross differences in nourishment, such as in Indian or African races, can diet really explain variations in physical and mental characteristics.

Such scientific cold water, however, does not deter many who claim that certain specific foods not only enhance physical fitness but improve mental acuity and sexual prowess as well. One old wives' tale had it, for example, that fish is good for the brain (although I've always liked the story of the young wife who, when related the tale by an old wife, replied: 'If fish are so clever, how come they get caught?'). The idea probably arose because fish, like the brain, is rich in phosphates. Fish is also, pound for pound, one of the best

sources of protein – but there is absolutely no connection between fish eating and brain power. The body is organised so that the brain gets top priority for the available nutrients and the rest of the body will go short before the brain is 'starved'. There is nothing you can eat to improve its efficiency.

And what about oysters and champagne for *l'amour*? Well, any successes are due to the breaking down of inhibitions by the alcohol rather than positive help from the bivalves. With the former the dosage is critical for, as Shakespeare noted, over-consumption is likely to increase the desire, but diminish the performance.

Even that universally believed old wives' tale that an apple a day keeps the doctor away seems to have little validity. Certainly the apple is a minor source of vitamin C but other fruits are far better: oranges, for example, are ten times richer. The apple's roughage was also supposed to keep you 'regular' but we know that the roughage from cereals and bran is far more effective. Nor is the apple a particularly good 'toothbrush', another virtue once assiduously promoted.

All that we can really say is that it has been cleared of one of its negative aspects. It used to be thought that apple pips, or other sharp objects, were the cause of appendicitis. This is not the case for many inflamed appendixes show no sign of any such offending irritant.

An astonishing variety of special foods for health and vigour have been recommended over the years – and often sold at high profit by the unscrupulous. There are more details about peculiar diets – like macrobiotics – and the so-called 'wonder foods' like sunflower seeds, molasses, honey and yoghurt, in Chapter Six.

Theology and Taboo

While the food faddists can undoubtedly make eating into a religion, religion over the millennia has certainly had plenty to say about eating. It was a very early belief that a man could suffer harm if his enemy got hold of the remains of a meal and cast spells on it – the Romans believed this too and took care to break the shells of eggs or snails they had eaten so that no magic could be wrought with them.

The corollary to this belief was that if you took food with a man you were his friend (were you to have cast a spell on any remains, you too would have been affected, through sympathetic magic) and ritual meals soon became established as important socio-religious ceremonies. Bread, in particular, assumed mystical significance but the implications of this, too, are discussed in detail in Chapter Six.

Certain foods are proscribed by religious sects – notably the Jewish shunning of pork. Other excellent sources of protein are taboo through social mores. The French seem to enjoy horseflesh, the British rather shudder at the thought; the Siamese as Hilaire Belloc tells us, eat puppy dogs but Europeans find the idea rather repulsive.

Because we 'civilised' races like to think that we are supremely rational creatures, finding our way through life's maze by logic, we tend to invent quasi-scientific reasons for why we eat what we do. Only primitive tribes, after all, are bound up with superstition.

Yet in reality our eating habits have little to do with logic and a lot with folklore. It has been suggested, for example, that Moses was acting as an inspired nutritionist in banning pork eating since pigs can be carriers of a parasitic disease *trichinosis*. But the connection between contaminated pork and the disease in man is a comparatively recent discovery and difficult to demonstrate without sophisticated equipment. Other races have enjoyed pork since the earliest times and Hippocrates commends it as providing more strength than other meats. The Chinese have used it since the Neolithic period and their sweet and sour sauce even dissolves pork bone, making available valuable calcium.

No, Moses' decision was most likely based on social custom: pigs cannot be herded over long distances and are therefore not popular with nomadic tribes. In their minds they come to be associated with the despised settled races and therefore to be shunned.

It appears to be a rather similar story with horseflesh too. Only France and Belgium seem to take to it in Europe although in Asia the horse is still often the animal of all trades, providing transport, hides, milk and meat. As Dr Pyke again points out in *Food and Society*: 'The most likely reason why Western dietitians feel a distaste for horse, in spite of the excellent quality of the protein of which it is mainly composed, has nothing at all to do with dietetics or for that matter with reason.'

'Horsemeat eating was at one time commonplace wherever horses were kept, from Mongolia all the way to Eastern Europe.

'Then, in the eighth century, Pope Gregory III ordered Boniface, his apostle to the Germans, to forbid the use of horseflesh by his Christian converts in order that they should show their separateness from the pagan tribes and vandals who ate wild horses and made a meal of horseflesh part of their pagan rites. And so there grew up in Christendom a belief that eating horses was wrong which persists to this day.'

The Moslems base their abhorrence of dogflesh on the basis that the canine species are unclean carrion eaters – and anyone who has seen the scavenging Pi dogs in the Middle East would be quick to agree. In Western Europe our reasons for not eating dog are more complex, bound up with the special relationship between man and dog in our society. Western man simply cannot eat his best friend. Yet in many countries, particularly in Africa, Polynesia and Asia, dog is a valuable and esteemed part of the diet, and has been for thousands of years. The Chinese, for example, bred a dog, the Chow, specially for food. And in parts of Africa, dogs are second in popularity only to pigs.

Entomophagy – or let them eat insects

I suppose that, given the right circumstances of hunger and food deprivation, most of us in the West could bring ourselves to eat mammal species like horse or dog, but what of insects? Could you stomach fried termite or five-inch long 'Witchetty grubs' as thick as your finger? It is certainly not my cup of tea, but entomophagy – the eating of insects – is still widely practised.

Fried termites are a West African delicacy and, at 561 Calories per 100 grams, have a high energy value. The Japanese enjoy a number of insect species, among them wasp maggots, silk worm larvae and grasshopper. Some grubs are even preserved in cans and sold over supermarket shelves.

The Witchetty grubs, thought to be the larvae of a big longicorn beetle, are a particular favourite of the Australian aborigine. Dug out from the roots of eucalyptus trees, the beetles are served lightly roasted.

It is normally the more primitive races that

continue to eat insects (although the modern Chinese use several kinds of beetles as confectionery) for as the nomadic hunter gradually settled to a stationary farming existence food supplies became more plentiful and foods such as leaves, berries and insects first became less highly prized and then, since they were not regularly or customarily eaten, became taboo.

There have been the occasional calls for a return to entomophagy. Among the latest was one from Australian zoologist V. B. Meyer-Rochow. Writing in *Search*, the journal of the Australian and New Zealand Association for the Advancement of Science, he said: 'Insects are extremely nutritious. They consist of easily-digestible proteins and fats and small but significant amounts of carbohydrates, minerals and vitamins.'

Earlier analyses of fried termites have shown that as well as those 561 Calories, 100 grams will provide 36 grams of protein and 44 of fat, placing them among the richest foods. Meyer-Rochow suggests that insect breeding programmes could provide even more nutritious foods. He is objective enough not to suggest that Europeans might be converted to entomophagy but suggests that its revival 'could ease the hazards of malnutrition in countries where the consumption of insects has only recently been given up'. They could be used, too, as a foodstuff for animals and poultry.

Salt and spice

We have been discussing above some gross differences in eating habits between races or ethnic groups. But there are, of course, considerable differences not only between 'national' cuisines but also in eating and cooking habits within the regions of any one country as well.

Such was not always the case. Indeed up until the late 16th century food would have been much of a muchness in, for example, most parts of Europe. Such standardisation was born more out of necessity than a lack of culinary imagination for the medieval chef's greatest problem was preserving his food through the long winters. (Most livestock had to be slaughtered before winter set in since feedstuffs were of poor quality and scanty and only a tiny minority of animals could be kept alive until spring.) So salting, drying and smoking to preserve meat were the order of the day. As Reay Tannahill says in her informative book, *Food in History*: 'Much medieval cooking, therefore, was specifically designed to make something interesting out of materials which, in unimaginative hands, would have had a dismal monotony.'

Salting was the preservation method of choice for most meats and fish and the medieval cook's first task was to get rid of the excess saltiness, by the tedious process of soaking the food in several

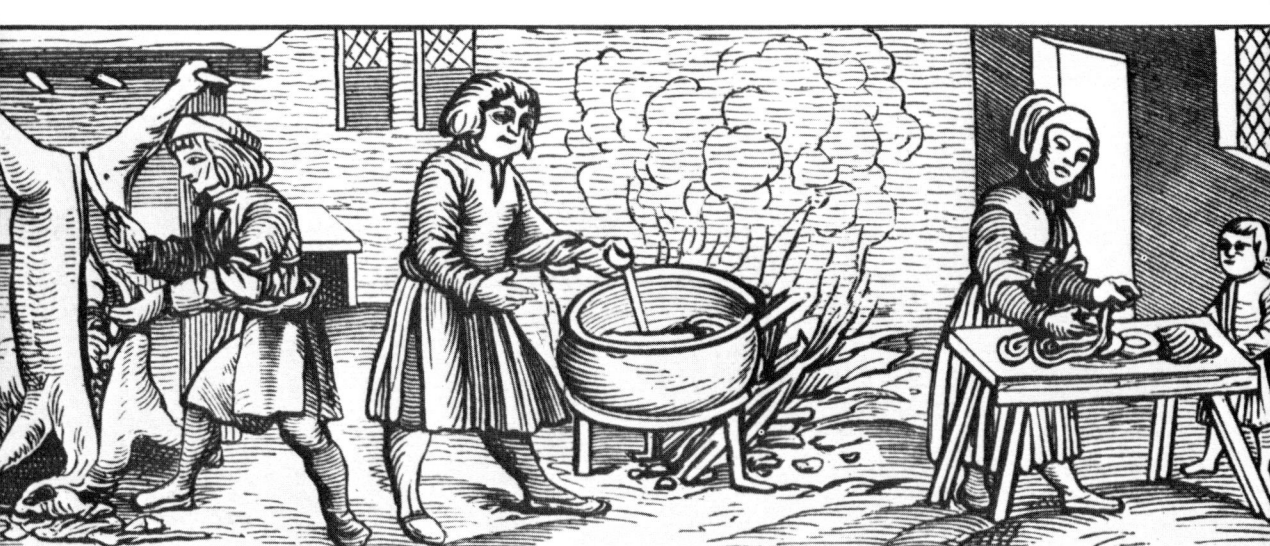

A scene in a mediaeval kitchen.

changes of fresh water or by cooking it with an accompaniment which would absorb the salt without itself becoming salty. Dried peas, beans, breadcrumbs and whole grain, all were used. In poorer households puréed beans and bacon were standard fare, but as Miss Tannahill points out 'the rich demanded something more enterprising. Their kitchen staffs did not neglect breadcrumbs and grain (which also had the property of thickening the mixture) but used in addition spices or fruit to offset any residual saltiness or creamy sauces to smooth it out.'

'Many medieval recipes look alarming at first, but the reader who blinks at the sight of pepper, ginger, cinnamon, saffron, cloves and mace all in one recipe would remain unmoved if "a pinch of mixed spice" were specified instead. Probably medieval cooks used a great deal more than a pinch, however – if only because the starchy ingredients which reduced saltiness also reduced the intensity of the spices themselves.'

It was only the rich who could afford much variety. The poor man's meal would be black bread plus a 'mess of pottage' from the stockpot, possibly followed by some cheese or a bowl of curds.

For the rich man's banquet there might be a number of courses, but these would be far different from today's ordered procession, being merely a haphazard collection of dishes, all placed on the table at the same time and from which one made a choice. Here's a 'monotonous' Parisian menu of 1393 collected by Reay Tannahill.

First course

Miniature pastries filled with codliver or beef marrow.
A cameline meat 'brewet' – pieces of meat in a thin cinnamon sauce.
Beef marrow fritters.
Eels in a thick spicy purée.
Loach in a cold green sauce, flavoured with spices and sage.
Large cuts of roast or boiled meat.
Salt water fish.

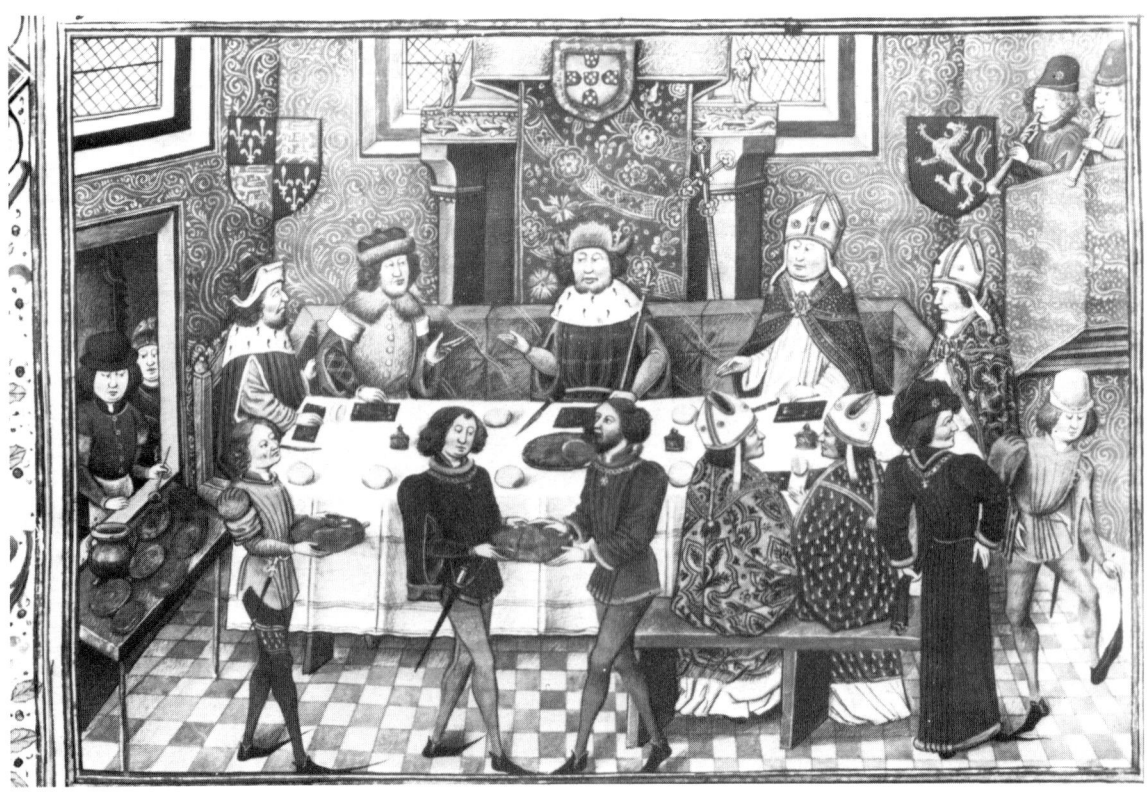

A royal banquet in the Middle Ages.

Second course

'The best roast as may be had.'
Freshwater fish.
Broth with bacon.
A meat tile – pieces of chicken or veal, sautéed and
served in a spiced sauce of pounded crayfish tails,
almonds and toasted bread.
Capon pasties and crisps.
Bream and eel pasties.
Blank Mang – the ancestor of blancmange –
shredded chicken blended with rice boiled in almond
milk and seasoned with sugar and, sometimes, salt.

Third course

Frumenty – a thick pudding of whole wheat grains
and almond milk, sometimes enriched with egg yolks
and coloured with saffron. The standard
accompaniment of:
Venison.
Lampreys with hot sauce.
Fritters.
Roast bream and darioles (pastry shells).
Sturgeon.
Jellies.

After this lot sweets and confections would be laid
out and either then or later spiced wines and wafers
were served and sometimes, dry whole spices 'to help
the digestion'.

A Gastronomic World Tour

It was the Italians who first broke out of the
medieval spice and sauce straitjacket. The loss of
the spice trade to the Portuguese and the political
turmoil of the early 16th century meant a scarcity
of spices and the Italians had therefore to rely on
local materials rather than flavourings for variety.
Meals may have been as long but individual dishes
tended to be simpler and served in a more
recognisable form. Of course, Italy's other great
contribution was pasta. Its origins are obscure but
the idea is thought to have been brought from
China by Marco Polo. Certainly the Chinese had
already developed the noodle centuries earlier and
this technique of processing wheat flour made a
welcome change from bread or flatcakes.

The Italian culinary revolution was exported to
France in the 16th century through Catherine de

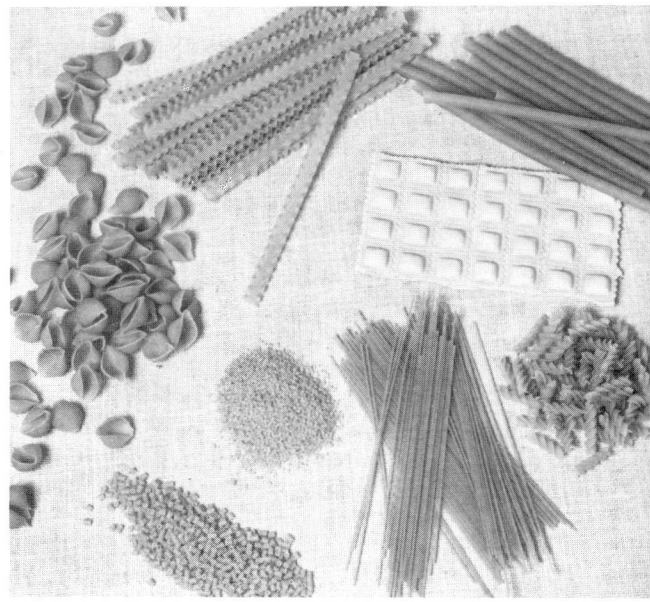

Varieties of pasta: spaghetti, macaroni,
conchiglie, ravioli, lasagne, canneloni etc.

Medici who left Florence to marry the heir to the
French throne in 1533 and Marie de Medici, the
bride of Henri IV at the end of the century. Not
only did these ladies take their own cooks but
introduced new vegetables, such as artichokes and
savoy cabbages, to the menu.

It took time for the new cooking to evolve but
by the middle of the 17th century Pierre François
de la Varenne was able to codify the Franco-
Italian cuisine. Reay Tannahill notes: 'La
Varenne frowned on spices and on thick meat and
almond mixtures. He recommended sauces based
on meat drippings combined merely with vinegar,
lemon juice (still an expensive luxury in France),
or verjuice (the juice of sour grapes or sometimes
of sorrel, green wheat or crab apples). He
provided 60 recipes for the formerly humble
egg. . .' France was well on the way to elevating
cooking to a true art – and scorning everyone
else's cuisines The stage was set for the coming of
the great chefs like Carême and Escoffier.

Most of the other citizens of Eastern and
Northern Europe (with the exception of the rich,
who sent their cooks to Paris for tuition), however,
rather scorned the French delicacy of touch and
sought what one English chef in 1710 described as
'substantial and wholesome plenty'. In an 18th
century gastronomic world tour, *Food in History*

describes Germany's staple diet as pork and sausage, cabbage, lentils, rye bread and beer. There was a thick soup at every meal and 'a fruit-stuffed goose on high days and holidays'. In Russia most of the population subsisted on black bread, soured dairy products, cabbage and *kasha* (made from buckwheat and either served as whole grain like a pilaff or made into a thin porridge). The Poles and the Hungarians inherited idiosyncratic items of diet from their numerous nomadic invaders, among them veal, pickled cabbage and capsicums. In the Low Countries much of the food was flat and heavy although the Dutch East India Company introduced a number of exotic fruits, some of which, like the plum, the cherry and the peach, came to be grown locally.

And what of England? Well, Miss Tannahill notes '. . . fruit was a feature only of the "tables of the great, and of a small number even among them"'. At the end of the seventeenth century, beef, mutton, fowls, pigs, rabbits and pigeons "infallibly" turned up, the mutton underdone and the beef salted for some days before being boiled and then served up besieged "with five or six heaps of cabbage, carrots, turnips or some other roots, well peppered and salted, and swimming in butter".

'Fifty years later the situation had improved a little. In 1748 a Swedish visitor remarked that "Englishmen understand almost better than any other people the art of properly roasting a large cut of meat". This, he went on, is not to be wondered at; because the art of cooking as practised by most Englishmen does not extend much beyond roast beef and plum pudding.'

'At their best – and their best was, no doubt, as rarely encountered in the 18th century as it is today – many of the dishes of Northern Europe could be superb, good filling food for a dank climate. But more often they must have been dull, tasteless, as lacking in food value as in savour.'

Across the Atlantic, on the Eastern seaboard of America, the 18th century colonists cooked and ate much as their European counterparts did. It was not until after the War of Independence and the Westward migration to open up the continent that 'pioneer' type dishes became popular – flapjack, bacon and beans, hash, pancakes and the like. The United States, of course, eventually became a great ethnic melting pot and a wide variety of national cuisines were assimilated. These included not only the way that the

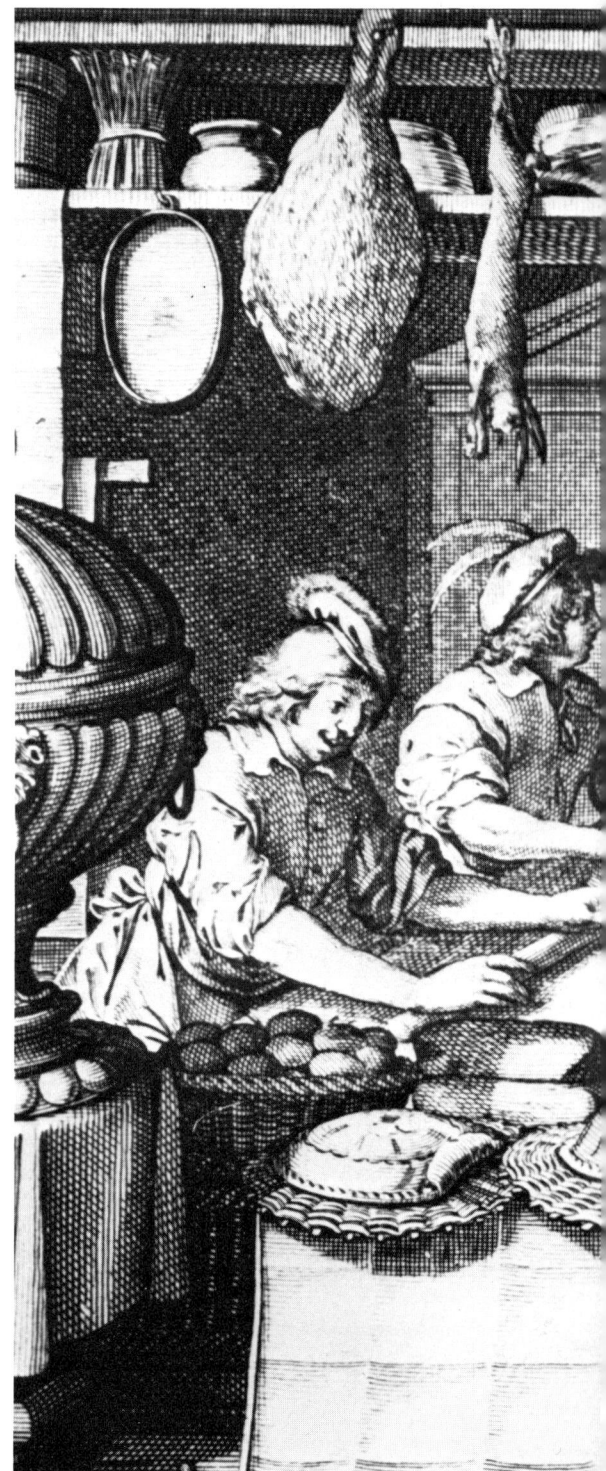

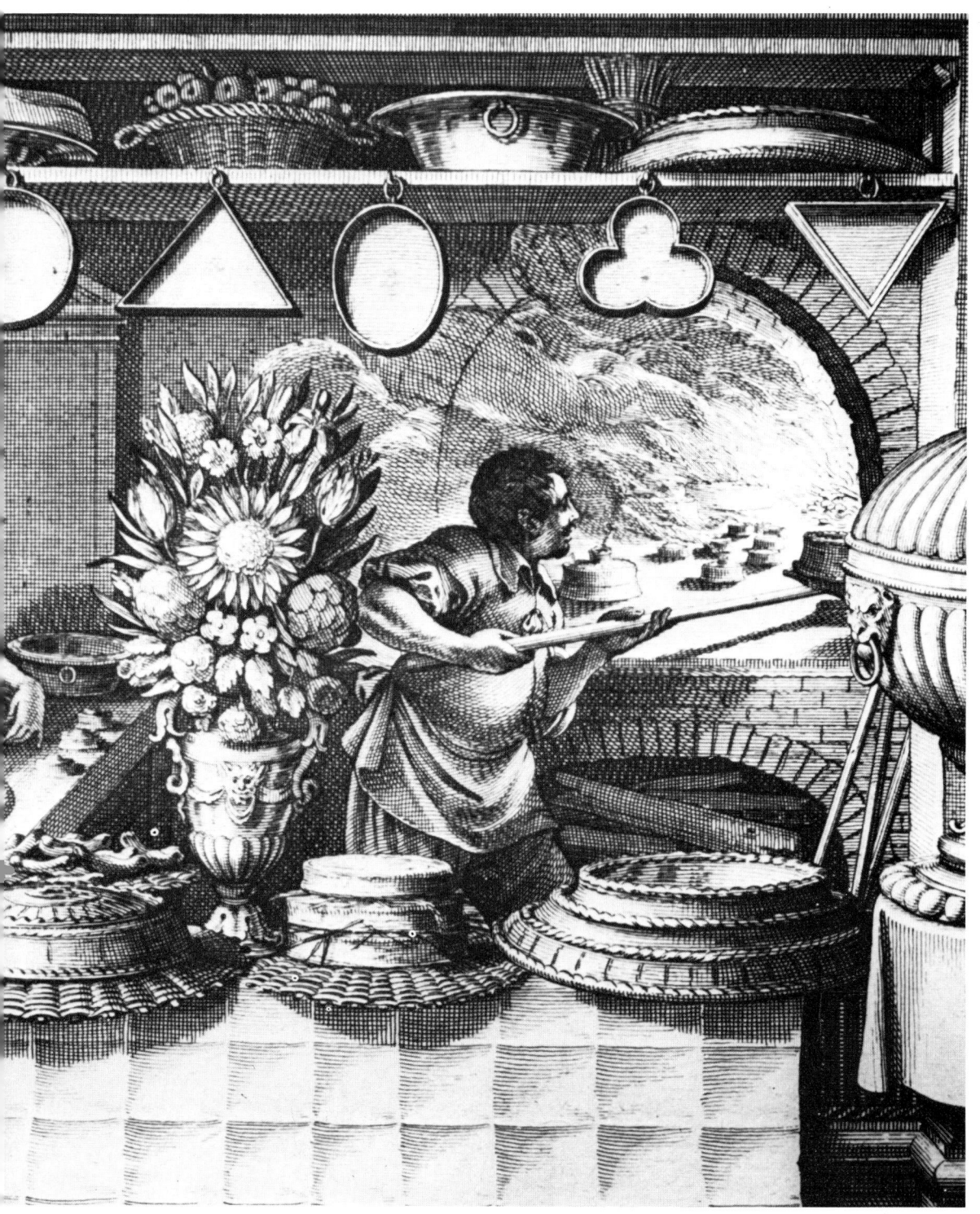

A 17th Century pastrycook.

Hamburgers and the Frankfurters served up their meat but also 'the English brought apple pie. The French introduced chowder (from *chaudière*, the fish kettle in which the dish was cooked). The Dutch took cookies (*koekjes*), coleslaw (*kool*: cabbage, and *sla*: salad) and waffles.'

South and Central American cuisine was greatly influenced by the Spanish conquest, at least as far as the rich were concerned. The Indians (those that survived) however, still subsisted on next to nothing and muted reality through chewing the coca leaf. There were also the gauchos – mounted vagrants who lived off the free-range cattle introduced by the Spaniards. Their diet had much in common with that of the nomads of Central Asia a thousand years previously.

Across the Pacific Ocean, in China, the average peasant of a couple of centuries ago ate little more than rice or noodles, supplemented by beans, curd, pork and a few vegetables. But the rich enjoyed a wonderful and, to Western eyes, weird diet which included birds' nest soup, sharks' fins and roasted snails. It was the dread of every Western visitor that they would be served red-cooked dog or stir-fried cat but by the end of the 19th century only the poorest ate such dishes.

Tea, of course, was the drink that China gave to the world. The Chinese had been making a careful infusion from the leaf of the tea bush for centuries before it was introduced into Europe. (It probably came from Japan to us, rather than directly from China.) The first public tea sale in Britain was in 1657 and 'the tea merchants claimed that the drink was the ultimate panacea – an infallible cure for migraine, drowsiness, apoplexy, lethargy, paralysis, vertigo, epilepsy, catarrh, colic, gallstones and consumption.' While Brooke Bond, Tetley or Typhoo might not today claim such sweeping benefits from 'the cup that cheers', Britons have certainly taken tea to their hearts. By the end of the 18th century we were consuming two pounds of it per head per annum, quite a consumption when one considers that a pound of tea can make nearly 300 cups. In the middle of this century consumption reached nearly ten pounds per person per year but in recent years there has been a steady decline in tea drinking: in 1974 our average per capita intake was 7·8 pounds.

The most far-reaching effect on Indian cooking came with the establishment of Muslim imperial power there in the 16th century. The followers of The Prophet had been drifting into the sub-continent for centuries before but as Miss Tannahill notes: 'At the court of the Moguls a new *haute cuisine* was introduced into India'. The cooking techniques originated in the splendid court of the Persian empire, at Isfahan: '. . . kebabs, pilaf (or pilau) dishes of rice with shredded meat, the technique of mixing fruit into flesh dishes, the use of almonds and almond milk, rose water, the garnishing of all kinds of food with thin strips of tissue beaten out of pure gold and silver – all these were absorbed into the Indian cuisine.

'Muslims were quite prepared to eat beef but their cuisine was based on mutton and chicken, and non-vegetarian Hindus were therefore able to adopt it without hesitation.'

Reay Tannahill ends her 18th century gastronomic grand tour in the Dark Continent. By this time coffee – which originated in Ethiopia – and chocolate – initially an American crop – were, apart from slaves, Africa's most important exports. The food of the natives was sparse and unenterprising: grains, legumes (peas, beans etc.), sour milk and occasionally beef, formed the basic diet.

As *Food in History* says: 'Ending his Grand Tour on the borders of unknown Africa, the travelling gastronome of the eighteenth century would have had at least one salutary lesson driven home to him – that cooking is an art only when food is consistently plentiful. When shortages are part of everyday life, filling the stomach is the only art.'

Eating today

That statement is as true of today as it was of 200 years ago. Certainly the revolutions of the last two centuries – in politics, economics, science, agriculture and transport – have gone a long way in increasing food supplies, enabling a wider distribution and ensuring a fairer share out of what is available. But for many millions of people, probably more numerically than ever before because of the population explosion, the diet is little more than a subsistence one.

For the rich nations cooking has become internationalised. In London or New York, for example, one can find restaurants of almost every nationality. The British housewife may serve her family dishes which originated in Italy, Hungary, America or China and excite little comment. And she may regularly prepare such dishes straight out of a packet.

The World Atlas of Food lists more than 500 recipes of specialists' dishes from all parts of the world. A glance at this atlas might lead one to suppose that the inhabitants of all the corners of the globe eat rather well. But the fact is that in many places the exotic dishes so mouth-wateringly described are seldom seen except on high days and holidays and even then only by the better off. For the poor of the 20th century, just as for the poor of the 18th century, variety in cooking is a seldom-enjoyed luxury.

For the vast majority of people on planet Earth 90 per cent of their diet consists of one of the three basic cereals – maize, wheat or rice – which are topped up with legumes and the occasional portion of animal protein. There is little time or concern for gastronomy. (The problems of feeding the world are discussed in detail in Chapter Seven.)

On the other side of the coin, the dietary difficulties in the developed nations spring more from over-consumption than from undernourishment. Most of us are simply eating too much food, or too much of the wrong type of food. We shall be looking at the potential dangers of this over-indulgence in Chapter Five.

But whether we are condemned to a diet, day in day out, of rice and beans or something similar, or whether we are able to gorge ourselves on pâté de fois gras avec truffles, Tournedos Henri IV and strawberries and cream, whatever we eat is very rapidly converted by our bodies to a few basic chemicals. We do, literally, very quickly become what we have eaten . . . as we shall see in the next chapter.

2 The whys and whats of eating

'The whole of nature is a conjugation of the verb to eat, in the active and passive.'

William Ralph Inge, 'Outspoken Essays'.

'All flesh is grass.'

Isaiah, Chapter 40, verse 6.

'The zebra is making grass fit for lions to eat, and the lion is producing meat fit for vultures to eat, and all three are producing food fit for the bacteria to consume eventually.'

Anthony Smith, 'The Body'.

'It's a very odd thing –
As odd as can be –
That whatever Miss T. eats
Turns into Miss T.'

Walter de la Mare.

One hundred pounds weight of oxygen and 28 of carbon. Fifteen lbs of hydrogen, 4·6 of nitrogen, 2·3 of calcium and 1·6 of phosphorus. . .

Eight and a half *ounces* of potassium, six of sulphur, 3·7 each of sodium and chlorine, 1·2 of magnesium and 0·15 of iron. . .

Some 1·9 *grams* of zinc, 0·2 of copper, 0·02 of manganese and 0·015 grams of molybdenum. . .

Even smaller amounts of selenium and cobalt and only the merest traces of one or two other elements. . .

Reduced to elemental essentials – chemically at least – that's what you are. It is all rather unimpressive, and even in these inflationary times such chemicals could be purchased for no more than a few pounds.

Of course, as with a Stradivarius violin or a Rembrandt self-portrait, it is not so much what you are made of that counts, but the way you are put together.

The complexities of our bodies are such that even today we are still unsure about much of the mechanics, even although we are rapidly unravelling many of the mysteries of the complicated interlocking biochemical reactions constantly going on within us all. Nonetheless we do have a basic understanding now of what we are and why and what we need to eat.

The human body is made up of millions upon millions of microscopic cells, with many different types of function. Some are joined to give the body structure, shape and motive power – as bones, skin, muscle and sinew. Others are grouped in vital internal organs, such as heart, lungs, stomach, intestines, liver and kidneys, or in essential chemical factories called glands. Some have specialised to form the sense organs like eyes and ears; yet others link up as nerve cells within the brain itself and in the network of nerve pathways to transmit sensations to the brain and receive instructions from it. There are scores of other types of cells, too.

Nature's 'building blocks'

But however specialised any body cell may be, its

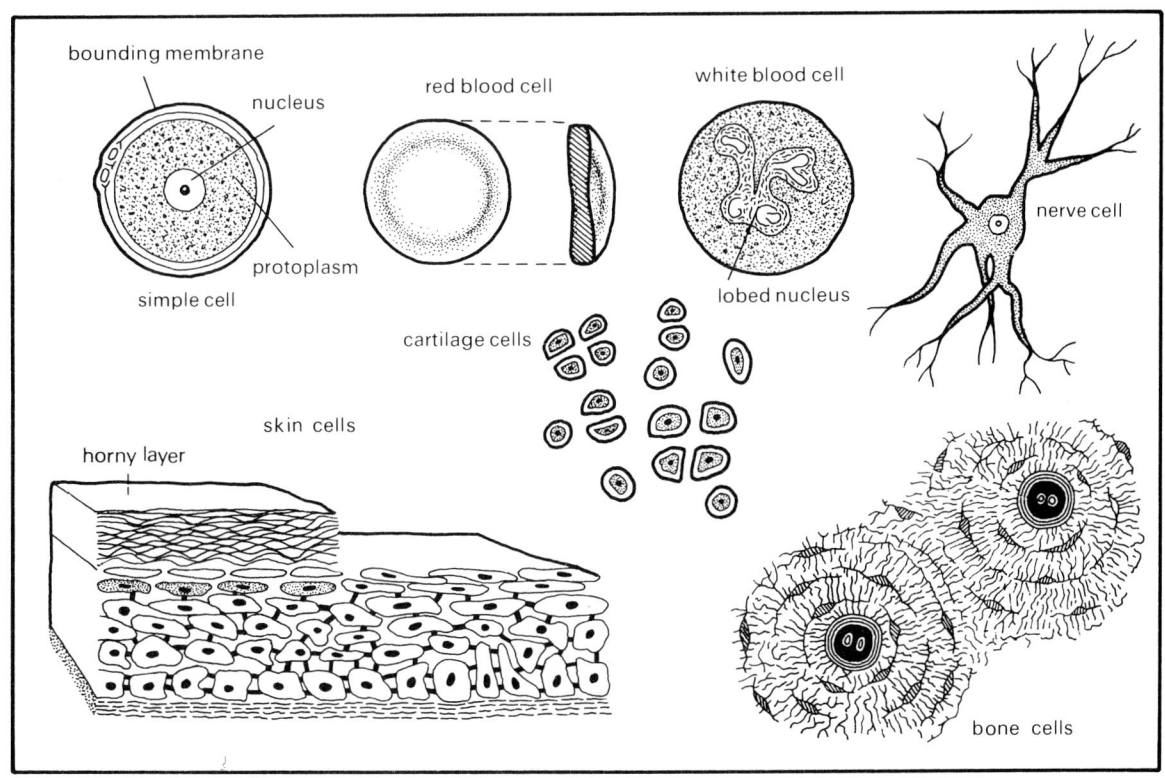

Some of the varied cell types found in the body.

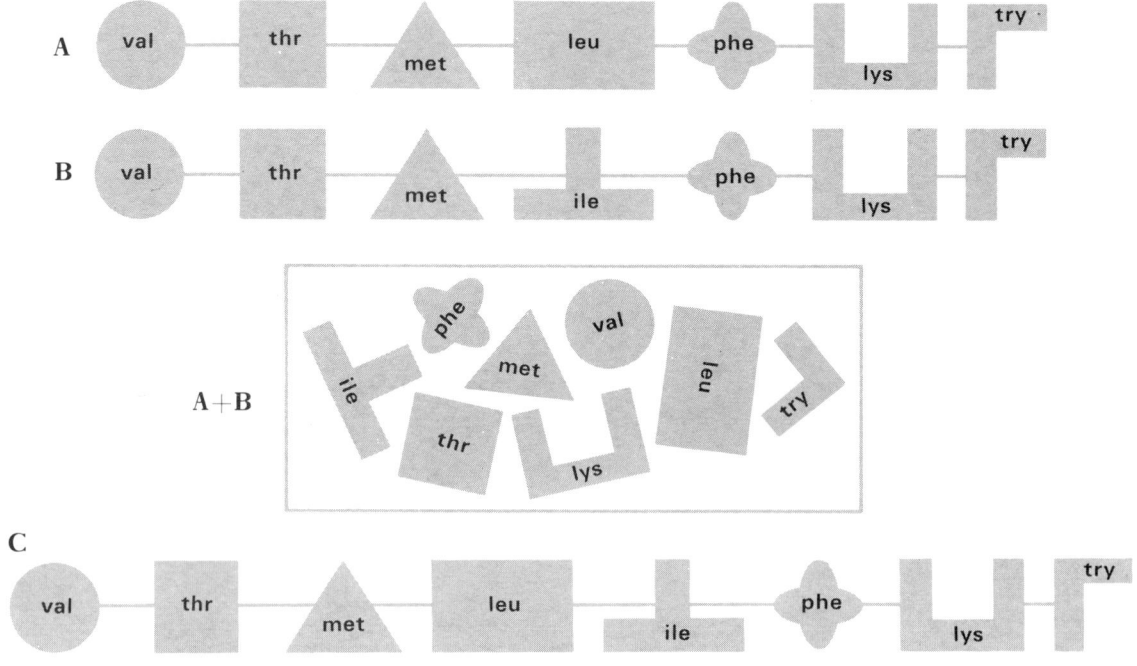

Protein chains are digested, broken down, then reconstructed to suit the body's needs. See page 33.

fundamental components will be various long and intricate chemical chains called proteins. These are the true 'building blocks' of all living matter and every living thing – man, mouse or oak tree – shares a common capacity in being able to put together proteins.

They are constructed by linking together, in all manner of orders, shapes and convolutions, other chemicals known as amino-acids. Hundreds of amino-acids may go to make one protein chain, and they may be combined in so many ways that the number of different proteins that could be constructed must be almost infinite.

What makes the difference between man, mouse and oak tree is almost exclusively the difference in the proteins they are able to make, for the other components of living material vary little from species to species.

The chemical blueprints for protein manufacture are locked in the genes, those 'packets of inheritance' that are passed on from generation to generation and are present in the nucleus of every living cell.

Man and the animals, however, have a basic protein manufacturing problem: they cannot build up all their complicated protein chains from scratch, from the basic chemical elements of

which they are composed. Were we to give a baby the right proportions of all those elements mentioned at the beginning of the chapter, there is simply no way that he could put them all together correctly.

Plants, on the other hand, *do* have this do-it-yourself protein-making capacity. They synthesise their proteins by taking carbon dioxide from the air and water, with many mineral substances dissolved in it, from the soil. The motive power for this operation is the light energy supplied by the sun – and the process is known as *photosynthesis.*

Not sharing such a capacity, animals and man have to obtain their protein, directly or indirectly, from plants. All flesh, as the Bible says, truly is grass. Some animals, like the cow or Anthony Smith's zebra, quoted at the beginning of this chapter, process the plant protein directly. Others, like the lion and ourselves, are another link further along on the 'food chain'.

When we digest the proteins in our food, they are slowly broken down into their amino-acid components, ready for re-assembly into our own types of protein, according to the instructions in those genetic blueprints.

So, the first answer to the question 'why do we

eat?' is: we eat to obtain the basic raw materials for protein manufacture, essential for building new body cells and for replacing or repairing old or damaged ones.

Unlocking the energy of the sun

But to carry out its myriad processes, the body needs far more than a supply of raw materials. For maximum efficiency, the temperature of the operation has got to be just right – and we need a source of power or energy to keep everything moving, from the beating of the heart to the internal activities of the smallest cell.

Once again the plant kingdom has the edge on man and the other animals: vegetation obtains its motive power from the sun. When we eat to obtain energy, what we are doing is unlocking this solar power, stored by plants rather as a battery stores electricity. Sometimes we obtain energy directly, by eating the plants themselves, and sometimes indirectly, by eating the animals that have eaten plants. The energy is released from the food by a process rather like burning (except that there is no flame) in which food is oxidised by body cells, using the oxygen we breathe in through our lungs.

Different foods, of course, have different energy-giving potentials and the food scientists have developed a system for assessing the amount of energy we can get from our food, the amount we use in various activities, and the amount we need when we are merely 'ticking over' during rest.

The way we do it is to measure the heat that would be given off *if* all our food was burned. Such 'heat energy' is equivalent to the energy we unlock from food within our bodies, some of which we use to power body processes, but much of which is actually dissipated as heat.

The unit of measurement is called the *Calorie*, with a capital *C*. You probably came across calories – with a lower case c – at school. That was the amount of heat needed to raise the temperature of one gram of water by one degree centigrade. The food scientists' Calorie ought technically to be called a *kilo*calorie since it is a

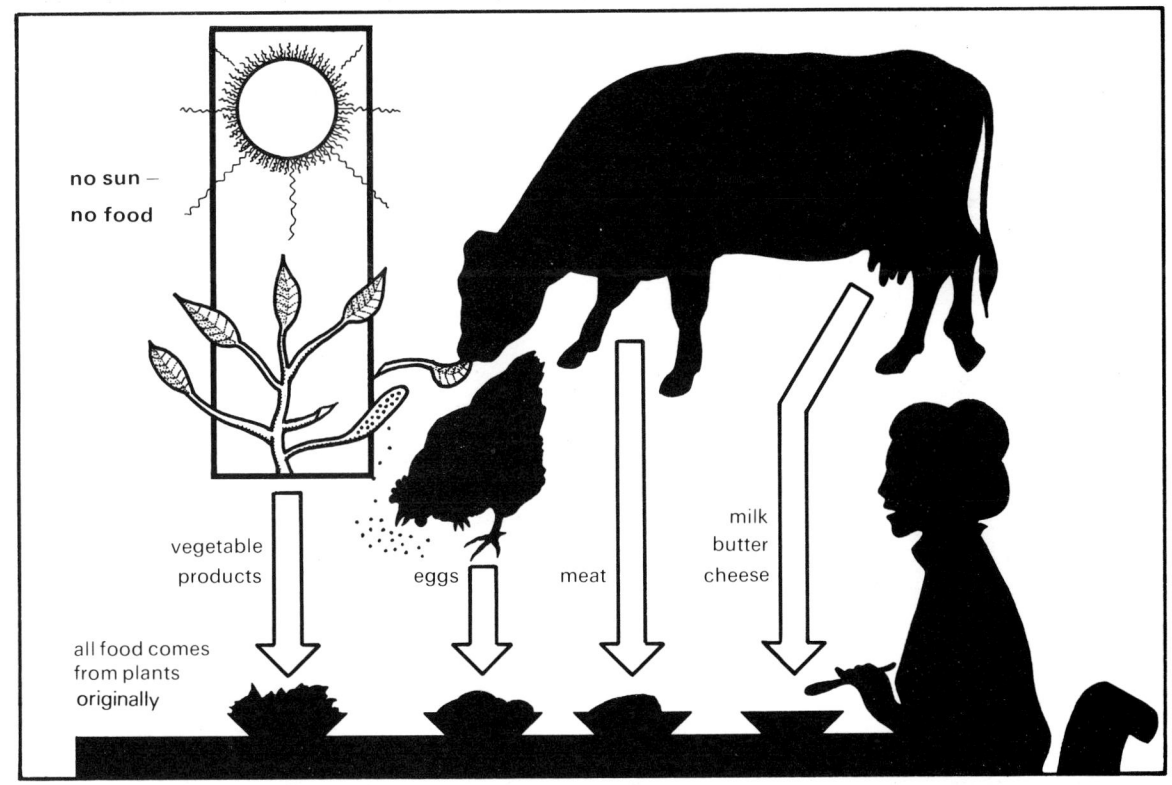

no sun –
no food

vegetable
products

eggs

meat

milk
butter
cheese

all food comes
from plants
originally

The basis of life: sunlight on plants. All animal life depends on this reaction.

thousand times bigger unit: it is the heat needed to raise the temperature of one *kilo*gram of water by one centigrade degree.

Not content with their calorific ambiguity, the food scientists now seem bent on fresh confusion by threatening to switch to the metric system, where energy is measured in *joules*.

I quote from one recent reference book: 'A thousand kilocalories (or Calories) is equivalent to 4·186 million joules, or 4·186 *megajoules* (MJ). One megajoule may be defined as the amount of heat needed to raise the temperature of approximately 239 kilograms of water by one degree centigrade'. One *kilo*joule is 1000 joules.

Well, we may be flying in the face of scientific so-called progress but in this book we will be sticking to Calories and letting the kilojoules take care of themselves. Those who wish to convert can conveniently multiply Calories by 4·1 and call the result kilojoules.

Some types of food, as we shall see later, have more energy locked in them that others.

One tenth of a horsepower

But how much energy do we require? Even when we are at rest, of course, many body processes are automatically at work. It is not just relatively large 'physical' processes like heart beat and breathing, nor the activities of internal organs, but also thousands of chemical reactions between cells and within the cells themselves. All these body chemical changes are known as *metabolism*, which

Getting up to date on energy measurement

1 Food energy is usually measured in **Calories (Cal.)**. The measure *used* to be cal. (small c), until nutritionists decided to multiply by 1000.
So now:

2 1 *C*alorie = 1000 calories (now out of use).

3 But some people call a Calorie a *kilo*calorie because it equals 1000 (kilo) old calories.
So now:
1 Calorie (Cal.) = 1000 calories *or* 1 kilocalorie (kcal.).

5 But even keener reformists now want to measure *all* energy in *joules* (J).
So now:

6 1 kcal (Calorie or kilocalorie) = 4·184 kJ (Kilojoules)

7 For reference,
1 kcal (or **1 Cal.**) *is the heat needed to warm 1 kilogram of water by 1 degree centigrade.*

can be regarded as having two parts: *catabolism*, the breakdown of large unmanageable molecules into smaller components – such as proteins into amino-acids; and *anabolism*, the reconstruction of large molecules.

The rate at which these processes continue is known as the *basal metabolic rate*. If a man of average build spent all day simply lying around he would need some 1500 to 1700 Calories, just to keep his body functioning. This is equivalent to some 80 watts in electrical terms or, if you are mechanically-minded, to about one-tenth of a horsepower. Put another way, the 'ticking over' energy used could heat 15 to 17 litres of ice-cold water to boiling point. That's enough for about 100 cups of steaming tea.

Your basal metabolic rate is more or less proportional to the surface area of your skin, although there are marked variations from the average and a variety of factors which can affect it both permanently and temporarily. It changes, for example, with age, increasing until we are around 25 years old and decreasing from about 35 onwards. Women in general have a lower basal metabolic rate than men. It rises after meals and falls during sleep. Exercise, as well as burning up Calories to meet increased energy demands, also increases the metabolic rate. Illness, emotional disturbance and certain drugs can all interfere with the body's 'tick over' speed. In a fever, for instance, the rate may be doubled or even trebled as the body needs heat to replace that lost by sweating.

Any physical activity obviously adds extra energy requirements to those needed to maintain the basal metabolic rate. Once you decide to get up, wash, walk to the station or shops, work at your office desk or do the household chores, you can add on another 1000 or 1200 Calories per day. And the more strenuous your exertion, the more energy you require. The basal rate is about 70 Calories an hour: running needs energy at an extra 600 Calories an hour; bicycling, some 360, and digging the garden demands another 350 or so Calories every hour.

There is no universal agreement on the standard daily Calorie requirements for people of different sexes and different occupations. Indeed, it sometimes seems as if every country and international agency uses their own standard. Bearing in mind the fluctuations from the average, any set of tables must be approached with care and used as a guide rather than a directive. Reproduced below, however, are the tables most often used in Britain.

It can be seen that the average man requires some 2700 to 3000 Calories a day while the average woman can manage with some 2200 to 2500.

So the second answer to the question 'why do we eat?' is that we eat to provide energy for body processes and to maintain body temperature.

Energy needed for everyday activities

Activity	Calories per minute
sitting still	1·4
standing still	1·7
washing \ dressing /	3·5
slow walking	3·0
fast walking	5·0
walking up and down stairs (average)	9·0
Light work assembly bricklaying domestic golf	2·5–4·9
Moderate work farm labour tennis dancing	5·0–7·4
Heavy work mining \ football /	7·5–9·0
lumbering \ steelwork /	10·0 or more

Activity	Time		Day's total Calories
Sleeping	8 hours		500
Work sitting	5 hrs (1·5 Cal. per min.)	450	
standing \ walking /	3 hrs (2·5 Cal. per min.)	450	900
Other activities washing \ dressing /	1 hr (3·5 Cal. per min.)	210	
walking	1 hr (4·2 Cal. per min.)	250	
sitting	4 hr (1·4 Cal. per min.)	340	
washing up	½ hr (1·7 Cal. per min.)	50	
gardening	1½ hr (5·0 Cal. per min.)	450	1,300
			2,700

So he needs to eat food providing about the same amount. For most *women* the total energy output is about 2,200 Cal. per day.

More essential supplies

Until the early years of this century it was thought that as long as anyone ate enough energy-giving foods and took in enough protein, he would be strong and healthy. It is not so. Many of the body's chemical processes will seize up without an adequate supply of a number of essential nutrients, which we generally describe as vitamins and minerals. We will look at the minerals first.

Although proteins are the basic building blocks of living cells, these all require additional raw materials to enable them to carry out their specialised tasks. Bone, for example, is basically a network of protein fibres made rigid with mineral salts (mostly calcium phosphates) deposited among them. Since bone tissue is constantly being absorbed and recreated, we must take in adequate supplies of *calcium* and *phosphorus* compounds to keep it healthy. And when bones – and teeth, which are similar structures – are growing, good supplies are doubly important.

Another essential mineral is *iron*, for the metal is a vital constituent of the red pigment in the blood called *haemoglobin*. This chemical is 'hungry' for oxygen and as the blood passes the tiny air sacs at the end of our lungs it grabs molecules of the life-giving gas for transportation to the body's cells. Without sufficient iron in the diet, people become anaemic – they become listless, look pale and may suffer slight fever and headache. Although the body usually conserves iron very well, we are losing a little through our skins all the time (about one milligram a day) and this needs to be continually replaced.

Iodine is vital too, in the make up of a hormone – one of the body's messengers – called *thyroxine*, which regulates the rate of chemical reactions in the body, speeding up the release of energy in cells, for example, when strenuous work or exercise demands it. Thyroxine is essential, too, for normal physical and mental growth and development. Yet, vital as it is, we only have about 0·025 grams of iodine in our bodies and our daily requirement is some 0·00005 grams, or slightly more than a millionth of an ounce.

The minerals you need

Mineral	What it does	Which foods
Calcium	Builds bones and teeth	Milk, cheese, bread
Iron	Needed for blood	Liver, kidney
Sodium	Maintains fluid balance	Salt, bacon, cornflakes, cheese, prunes, sprouts, mushrooms, cauliflower
Phosphorus	Needed for bones, teeth, hair, fingernails	Most
Iodine	Used by thyroid gland	Sea-food, most normally grown vegetables. A few areas have iodine-deficient soil and water, and goitre results if iodine is not added to diet.

Other essential supplies include *sodium chloride*, common salt, found mainly in body fluids; *potassium*, needed within body cells, and *magnesium* which, like calcium, is found in bones. *Chlorine*, *bromine* and *fluorine* are needed, too, as are *copper*, *cobalt*, *zinc*, *manganese* and *molybdenum*. All in all our bodies contain less than a gram (0·0353 ounces) of the last five, but without them we would die. They are essential in the manufacture of enzymes, the catalysts which trigger off chemical reactions within the body. Those, then, are the vital minerals. We need also, however, to take in certain compounds which the body requires but cannot put together on its own. These are called vitamins and most of them are needed to promote chemical reactions within the body.

'Accessory food factors' – the 'vital amines'

One of the nicest analogies about vitamins comes from Dr Peter Wingate, in the *Penguin Medical Encyclopaedia*. He says that one's body system 'might be compared with the workshop of a versatile carpenter. He can fashion all the parts of a piece of furniture and makes his own glues and varnishes. But he cannot make screws; these he must buy ready-made. If he cannot buy screws he turns out rickety furniture held together only with glue and nails.

'So it is with vitamins. One may survive without them, but not in good health, and not for the full span.'

One of the extraordinary facts about vitamins is just how little we need of some of them. We can manage perfectly well on less than an ounce of thiamine (vitamin B_1) *in our whole lifetime*, as long as we get our microscopic supplies regularly.

But without the vitamins, even in such tiny amounts, the body systems begin to seize up, precipitating what are called deficiency diseases. Some such diseases, although not their cause, have been known for ages: beri-beri, rickets, scurvy.

Every schoolboy knows how sailors learned the value of fresh fruits for combatting scurvy in the 18th century and how British seamen earned the epithet 'limeys' because of their predeliction for citrus fruits (which are rich in vitamin C). By the end of the 19th century beri-beri was shown to have dietary links and children with rickets were given cod liver oil, although again, as with the fruit, nobody knew *why* it worked.

It was not until 1906 that Sir Frederick Gowland Hopkins suggested that such diseases might be due to a lack of 'accessory food factors' and in 1911 another expert Casimir Funk used the word 'vitamine' to describe such a factor, amalgamating the words 'vital' and 'amine' (a type of chemical). It was soon established that although they certainly were vital, few of them were amines – and the nutrionists disguised their error by dropping the final 'e'.

They also tied themselves up in knots as far as labelling the vitamins was concerned. The alphabetical listing of each new discovery was rather upset by subsequent discoveries. It was found, for example, that vitamin B was in fact a group of vitamins, which were labelled B_1, B_2 and so on. Today, although you will come across vitamins E and K, you will hear next to nothing about vitamins F, G, H, I and J. Where are they now? Well, H for example, was shown soon after

---

Notes to table on page 29

[1] Units used are quite different for each vitamin. The figures shown give an idea of proportion only.

[2] Also: Folic acid, B_{12}, Pyridoxine, Pantothenic acid, Biotin.

[3] White bread has nicotinic acid *added* by law.

Which foods have which vitamins?

Vitamin	Action in body	Food source	[1]units per oz
A	Needed for child growth. Needed for healthy vision. Protects surface of eye and lining of throat and bronchial tubes. *Too much is harmful.*	Fish liver oil	255,000
		Butter	282
		Margarine	255
		Cheese	120
		Eggs	85
		Carrots	567
		Spinach	284
		Watercress	142
D	Proper development of bones. *Partly provided by action of sunlight on skin.*	Codliver oil	61·66
		Herring	6·38
		Salmon (canned)	3·54
		Margarine	2·27
		Eggs	0·36
		Butter	0·36
E	Required in small amounts for body chemistry.	Vegetable oils	
		Wheat germ	small amounts
		Eggs	
		some Margarines	
B group[2]			
1 Thiamine	Needed for steady release of energy from carbohydrates in the organs.	Dried Yeast	5·22
		Pork	1·00
		Peas	0·32
		Wholemeal bread	0·07
		White bread[3]	0·05
		Potatoes	0·03
		Beef	0·02
2 Riboflavine	Necessary link in energy production.	Dried Yeast	1·04
		Liver	0·85
		Cheese	0·14
		Eggs	0·10
		Milk	0·04
3 Nicotinic acid	Necessary link in energy production.	Dried Yeast	17·8
		Liver	4·9
		Beef	2·2
		White fish	1·7
		Peas	1·0
		Wholemeal bread	0·5
		White bread[3]	0·7
		Potatoes	0·5
		Milk	0·3
C	Healthy growth and repair of tissues. Prevention of *scurvy*. *Quantities vary greatly according to season and freshness.*	Rose-hips	700
		Blackcurrants	57
		Brussels sprouts (raw)	28
		Cabbage (raw)	17
		Citrus fruit	14
		Potatoes (raw)	
		new	9
		Oct/Nov	6
		Jan/Feb	4
		March onwards	3
		Tomatoes	6
		Lettuce	4
		Apples	
		Plums	1
		Pears	

its discovery to be identical with Biotin, a vitamin in the B complex.

To sort out the mess, the trend now is to call them all by their chemical names, but it seems that the idea of 'vitamin C' and so on is so ingrained in the public mind that changing the usage is going to be easier said than done.

There is also the problem of when is a vitamin not a vitamin? Most animals, for example, can manufacture their own vitamin C, so it is not an essential accessory food factor for them. On the other hand, were you to deprive rats of vitamin E, they would become sterile; but there's no conclusive evidence that humans need this vitamin at all.

In the public mind vitamins seem to have taken on the mantle of the magic elixir and people are consuming vast quantities of them in the belief that 'over-kill' will make them healthier and fitter. The evidence for such a belief is at best tentative and we'll be dealing with vitamania in a later chapter.

As far as deficiency diseases are concerned, lack of vitamin A (retinol) can lead to night-blindness, dry and inflamed eyes, bad skin and decreased resistance to infection. Long-term deficiency can lead to a disease called *xerophthalmia* and ultimately, to blindness. The B complex – and it really is complex – includes *thiamine* (B_1), *riboflavin* (B_2), *pyridoxine* (B_6), *cobalamin* (B_{12}), *nicotinic acid, biotin, pantothenic acid* and *folic acid*. The two diseases associated with B-group deficiency are beri-beri, mainly a lack of B_1, and pellagra, largely a lack of nicotinic acid. Probably no diet lacks B_{12} but pernicious anaemia results from an inability to assimilate it from food. Incidentally B_{12} is the only vitamin containing a metal atom, namely cobalt. Lack of B group vitamins can also affect the growth of children. Too little thiamine may lead to loss of appetite, fatigue, nervous irritability and a type of neuritis, or inflammation of the nerves.

Riboflavin lack also stunts growth, leads to tongue and mouth inflammation and a possible misting of the cornea.

Shortage of nicotinic acid may lead to rough skin, diarrhoea and in extreme cases mental disorders and derangement, and ultimately pellagra and death.

Vitamin C prevents scurvy, is essential for proper growth and helps wound healing. Vitamin D is necessary for the formation of healthy bone;

without it, rickets or in adults a similar disease, known as osteomalacia, may develop. Vitamin E, as we have seen, has not proved its value. Vitamin K is required for the formation of an enzyme called *thrombin* without which blood will not clot.

What is sometimes not realised is that vitamins taken to excess can in some instances be as dangerous as deficiency. In 1974, for example, a health food addict who drank six to eight pints of carrot juice – a rich source of vitamin A – every day, died by literally poisoning his liver with the substance. Excess vitamin D can be dangerous too.

One curious fact about vitamins is that there are no chemical similarities between the various types. They are simply, as one researcher has called them, 'the odds and ends of vitally needed materials'.

The third answer, then, to the question 'why do we eat?' is that we eat to provide essential chemicals – vitamins and minerals – for the body's internal processes.

Water, water everywhere

There is yet another important ingredient which is sometimes ignored by those writing or talking about diet – water. Without food a man could probably survive for some two months; without water he would be lucky to last as long as ten days.

Life on this planet, it seems, began in water and that liquid is by far the commonest component in our bodies: 60 per cent of the average man is water, and 50 per cent of the average woman. The difference is accounted for by body fat. A woman has proportionately more – it gives her a more rounded shape – and fat contains very little water.

No other substance plays as many roles in body processes as water. It is an ideal solvent: it can carry body chemicals from one place to another – either in solution or in suspension – without itself being changed. And it is very useful for cooling since it evaporates fairly easily at body temperatures but soaks up a considerable amount of heat while doing so.

The fatter you are, the less water you contain, but for a rough guide, a healthy nine-stone girl will be comprised of some 32 litres, or about six and a quarter gallons of water. An eleven-stone man will have 42 litres – or just over nine gallons – in his make up.

The blood itself is largely water. There are some three litres of *plasma*, the blood's liquid part, in the average person. Most of the nutrients from the food are absorbed into the blood through the walls of the small intestine, which actually have a surface area of some 100 square feet or five times that of the skin. Some chemicals can be transported directly to cells, others have first to be processed into useful forms by specialised 'factories' within the body, notably the liver and other glands.

The tiny capillaries at the ends of the blood vessel system and the walls of cells allow water, sugars, amino-acids and some other chemicals to seep through but they are impervious to big molecules, like the proteins themselves.

Through a process called *osmosis* the arterial capillaries (bringing blood *from* the heart) give up water, with all its nutrients, to the tissue fluid. The venous capillaries (at the beginning of the blood's journey *back* into the heart) with their lower pressure, take in water again, this time bringing with it waste products from the tissue fluid.

Within the cells themselves, every chemical reaction takes place in water.

We lose water from our bodies not only in the final expulsion of waste products and in its evaporation from the skin during the cooling process of perspiration, but also through our lungs every time we breathe out. All in all, the average housewife in a temperate climate, for example, will use up about $2\frac{1}{2}$ to 3 litres – between four and five pints – a day. Strenuous activity and hot conditions can mean that as much as ten litres of water a day can be lost through perspiration alone.

Fluid loss must be replaced otherwise the body systems begin inexorably to seize up, since all metabolic reactions take place in water. We do not have to take in the five pints or so directly, since most of the food we eat contains water too. Cooked lean meat, for example, contains 65 to 70 per cent water. (So two-thirds of an expensive steak in a restaurant is actually warm water.) Food usually provides about half our daily water needs.

Another 300 to 400 millilitres is a by-product of the food burning process. One curious aspect of this is that although fat contains no water, when it is burned up it produces more than twice as much water, gram for gram, as protein.

The average Briton probably needs to take in about one litre ($1\frac{3}{4}$ pints) of water directly – in tea, coffee, milk, soft drinks, beer, etc.

So the fourth and final answer to the question 'why do we eat (and drink)?' is that we do so to replenish water supplies, essential to the body machine.

What makes us eat?

The will to survive is the most basic of all inborn mechanisms – and since we must have both food and water for survival, we have instinctive cravings to seek out, and take in, both. We call these 'hunger' and 'thirst'.

Scientific experiments have shown that there are specific centres in the brain responsible for these desires and, equally important, for switching them off when we have taken in enough. They are located in a small but vital area deep within the centre of the brain called the *hypothalamus*.

When the 'hunger sites', for example, are stimulated, even by an artificial electric current, we have an overwhelming desire for food. But when the nearby 'satiety sites' receive nervous messages, we feel replete, no longer needing food.

Such mechanisms work very well in animals and, by all accounts, in primitive man too. You will seldom see a fat lion, or any wild animal. This is not because of lack of ample supplies of food. Rather the animal eats and drinks when it is hungry and thirsty, and when it has had enough, it stops.

Modern man has seriously perverted this eminently sensible in-built apparatus: he eats when he is not hungry and he drinks when he is not thirsty. He has done so by introducing another factor into the desire for food, which is best described as *appetite*.

Hunger is the sensation of emptiness resulting from abstinence from food. Appetite has two inter-related parts: the desire for food (and often a specific kind of food), and the sheer pleasure of the process of eating itself. Hunger is inborn, appetite is not; it is what the psychologists term a 'conditioned response', something that is learned.

Every newborn baby soon experiences hunger, but he has no appetite. The coaxing of his parents, his growing experience of the world about him, however, soon give him that desire for food unrelated to his body's needs.

And the techniques of mass advertising influence this appetite even further. It is important to realise that few, if any, food advertisements rely on catering for hunger. They are out to create an appetite for their products, a desire which in nutritional terms is very often totally illogical.

And extra food, beyond the baby's needs, does not supply extra energy. Invariably it forms fat, leading to extra weight with all its attendant health problems.

Of all the perversions of appetite, the most universal is a 'sweet tooth', a craving for sugar and sweetness. At best, our sugar intake is unnecessary as it is easily replaced by other foods. At worst, it is downright harmful, being implicated in a wide range of unhealthy conditions, from tooth decay to heart disease.

We will be returning to the vexed question of hunger and appetite later on, when we look at the sugar story and at the problems of obesity (Chapter Five).

Taking in the building materials

We have seen that there are four fundamental answers to the question: Why do we eat?, namely to obtain basic raw materials for protein manufacture, to provide energy, to take in essential vitamins and minerals and to preserve fluid levels.

The substances in our food which supply these needs – *proteins, carbohydrates, fats, vitamins* and *minerals* – are known as *nutrients*.

Now, human proteins are subtly different from, but related to other animal proteins. Plant proteins differ far more but they nonetheless contain amino-acid building blocks of use to us.

All in all, there are some twenty-two different types of amino-acids in animal proteins. (The *amino* part of the name comes from 'the *amino* group' – a combination of two hydrogen atoms and one nitrogen atom – NH_2. Amino-acid molecules also contain carbon atoms and acidic chemical groups. But just as most 'vitamines' are not actually amines, so most amino-acids are neutral in character [neither acid nor alkaline]. The early food scientists certainly seem to have had a hard time, one way and another.)

Amino-acids link together into complex, curling, convoluted chains of molecules, called *polypeptides*, which in turn are linked together to form the proteins.

In the process of digestion, animal and plant proteins taken in are broken down into their amino-acid constituent parts, ready for re-assembly into the variety of different kinds of proteins our bodies need.

Of the twenty-two or so different types of amino-acid, all but eight can in fact be created within the body from other amino-acids and simpler chemicals. Those eight, however, are absolutely vital components of any diet because without them we cannot assemble proteins necessary to maintain life. They are known as the *essential amino-acids*.

After the food proteins are broken down during digestion, the amino-acids circulate in the blood, from which they can be removed, as required, for cell repair, maintenance and growth. Surplus amino-acids are burned up for heat and energy.

The usefulness of food proteins to the body is measured as '*biological value*' – the better the proportions of essential amino-acids, the higher the biological value. It is not surprising that the highest of such values come from animal products, such as meat and fish themselves and milk, cheese and eggs. The lowest biological values are found in plant proteins, such as cereals or nuts, but there are a few striking exceptions to this rule: the best known is the soya bean, which contains all the essential amino-acids and is rapidly becoming one of the world's most important sources of protein – we will be hearing more about this remarkable bean in a later chapter (see page 124) but if you think you have never eaten it, look closely at packets and tins of food in your kitchen. You will be surprised how often soya bean flour occurs in the list of contents.

But even plants with lower biological values are of protein-building use to us, as supplements to the protein-rich meat and dairy products. In fact it is generally reckoned that in the ideal diet half

Protein content of some foods

Animal	grams per oz	Vegetable	grams per oz
Cheese	7·2	Peanuts	8·0
Haddock	4·5	Dried peas	6·1
Beef	4·2	White flour	2·8
Lamb	3·7	Wholemeal bread	2·7
Eggs	3·4	White bread	2·4
Milk	0·9	Baked beans	1·7
		Fresh peas	1·6

It is good sense to mix animal and vegetables proteins in your diet. They complement each other.

Your food must contain

Full name	Shortened to
Valine	val
Threonine	thr
Lysine	lys
Methionine	met
Leucine	leu
Isolencine	ile
Phenylalanine	phe
Tryptophan	try

Foods vary in their content of these amino acids. To be healthy you need a certain amount of each. The table below shows how some common foods vary in their content of the different essential amino acids.

Protein scores of some foods

Type of food (100=excellent)			ile	leu	lys	phe	met	thr	try	val
Meat and Fish	Egg	100	428	565	396	368	196	310	106	460
	Beef	83	332	515	540	256	154	275	*75	345
	Milk	80	402	628	497	334	190	272	*85	448
	Fish	70	317	474	549	231	178	283	*62	327
Cereals	Oats	79	302	436	*212	309	*84	192	*74	348
	Rice	72	322	535	*236	307	*142	241	*65	415
	Flour	47	*262	442	*126	322	*78	174	*69	262
	Maize	42	293	827	*179	284	*117	249	*38	327
Other Vegetables	Soya	73	333	484	395	309	*86	247	*86	328
	Pea	58	336	504	438	290	*77	230	*74	317
	Potato	56	*260	304	326	285	*87	237	*72	339
	Cassava	22	*118	*184	310	*133	*22	*136	131	144

*indicates levels below those required for health.

the protein intake should come from animal foods and half from plant foods. (Incidentally, the phrase 'a balanced diet' is often used in nutrition. It means simply a diet in which there is sufficient, but not too much, of all the nutrients the body requires.)

There is considerable debate raging at present about just how much protein we need. Certainly children need more to serve their growing bodies than do adults. But it seems as if once we have reached maturity we can manage perfectly well on two ounces a day – and probably even less. A *breakfast* of bacon, sausage and eggs could easily cover the *day's* protein needs. There will be more about the great protein debate in Chapter Seven.

The Calorie value of proteins is slightly higher than that of carbohydrates so any excess intake makes extra Calories available within the body. Happily, however, increased protein intake accelerates the rate at which the body burns up foods, so those extra Calories are likely to be burned rather than stored as fat.

Just as there are certain foods rich in essential amino-acids, so too some are excellent sources of the essential vitamins and minerals. Milk, for example, provides plenty of calcium and phosphorus; good sources of iron are liver, kidney, meat, eggs and a variety of vegetables and cereals; iodine is found in fish, shellfish, onions and watercress.

The tiny amounts of vitamins needed each day come from a wide variety of sources: dairy products, fruits, vegetables, meat, fat fish (like herrings and sardines), bread and flour. An ordinary balanced diet contains more than enough.

The proteins, vitamins and minerals are the body-building, protective and regulatory foods. Foods to be burned – the energy providers, are known as carbohydrates and fats.

The energy providers
The word 'carbohydrate' comes from the Latin for *coal* and the Greek for *water*. They are made up

c

One day's sample balanced diet for a woman doing normal work

Breakfast

Cornflakes	$\frac{1}{2}$ oz	Cpf/B
Milk	4 oz	cpf/ADBC
Sugar	$\frac{1}{4}$ oz	C/–
Boiled egg	2 oz	PF/ADB
Toast	2 oz	Cpf/B
Butter	$\frac{1}{2}$ oz	F/AD
Marmalade	$\frac{1}{2}$ oz	C/–
Tea		(no value)
Milk	2 oz	cpf/ADBC
Sugar	$\frac{1}{2}$ oz	C/–

Mid-morning

Coffee		(no value)
Milk	2 oz	cpf/ADBC
Sugar	$\frac{1}{4}$ oz	C/–

Lunch

Tomato Soup	6 oz	Cpf/ADB
Cheese salad:		
cheese	2 oz	Pf/ADB
lettuce	1 oz	cp/ABC
tomato	$2\frac{1}{2}$ oz	cp/ABC
beetroot	$1\frac{1}{2}$ oz	Cp/B
watercress	$\frac{1}{2}$ oz	cp/ABC
Bread	2 oz	Cpf/B
Butter	$\frac{1}{2}$ oz	F/AD
Fruit Yoghourt	5 oz	CPf/AB
Coffee		(no value)
Milk	2 oz	cpf/ADBC
Sugar	$\frac{1}{4}$ oz	C/–

Afternoon

Tea		(no value)
Milk	2 oz	cpf/ADBC
Sugar	$\frac{1}{2}$ oz	C/–

Supper

Roast chicken	3 oz	Pf/b
Peas	3 oz	Cp/ABC
Brussels sprouts	3 oz	cp/ABC
Roast potatoes	4 oz	Cpf/BC
Canned Peaches	4 oz	Cp/ABC
Single Cream	2 oz	CpF/ADB

Key

C=carbohydrate
P=protein
F=fat
(Capital letter indicates more than small letter)
Letters after / indicate vitamins.
eg: Cpf/ADB meant plenty of carbohydrate, some protein and fat, vitamins A, D and B.

This day's food intake provides the following:

Components of days intake	Value	Remarks
Energy	2,224 Cal.	Most women need about 2,200 Cal.
Protein	89·8 g.	More than adequate. Most women need about 55 g. protein.
Calcium	1,461 mg.	Plenty. Recommended 500 mg.
Iron	13·1 mg.	Approx. 12 mg. recommended.
Vitamin A	1,367	Adequate. 750 recommended.
Vitamin D	1·61	Less than recommended, but probably sufficient, particularly if exposed to sun.
Thiamine	1·14 mg.	Enough. 0·9 mg. recommended.
Riboflavine	2·07 mg.	Enough. 1·3 mg. recommended.
Nicotinic acid	32·9	More than adequate. Approx. 15 mg. recommended.
Vitamin C	93 mg.	30 mg. recommended.

of carbon, hydrogen and oxygen atoms and the proportions of hydrogen and oxygen are the same as those in water. There are a few exceptions, but carbohydrates are almost entirely plant products, made from carbon dioxide and water, the motive power for the process coming from the sun's energy. The simplest carbohydrates, called *monosaccharides* (or single sugars) are the three sugars: *glucose, fructose* and *galactose.* All other carbohydrates are built up of combinations of monosaccharide units, just as different proteins are varying arrangements of amino-acids. *Sucrose*, for example, is a 'double sugar', being a combination of glucose and fructose.

Those sugar names, incidentally, are fairly straightforward. Glucose, for instance, is 'grape sugar', based on the Greek *glykys*, for sweet. Fructose (Latin, *fructus*, fruit) is 'fruit sugar'. Sucrose comes simply from the French *sucre*. Galactose and lactose are both 'milk sugars' (Latin *lactis* and Greek *galactos*) and *maltose* (English, malt) is malt sugar. This last is actually a double sugar, or *disaccharide*, like sucrose, but

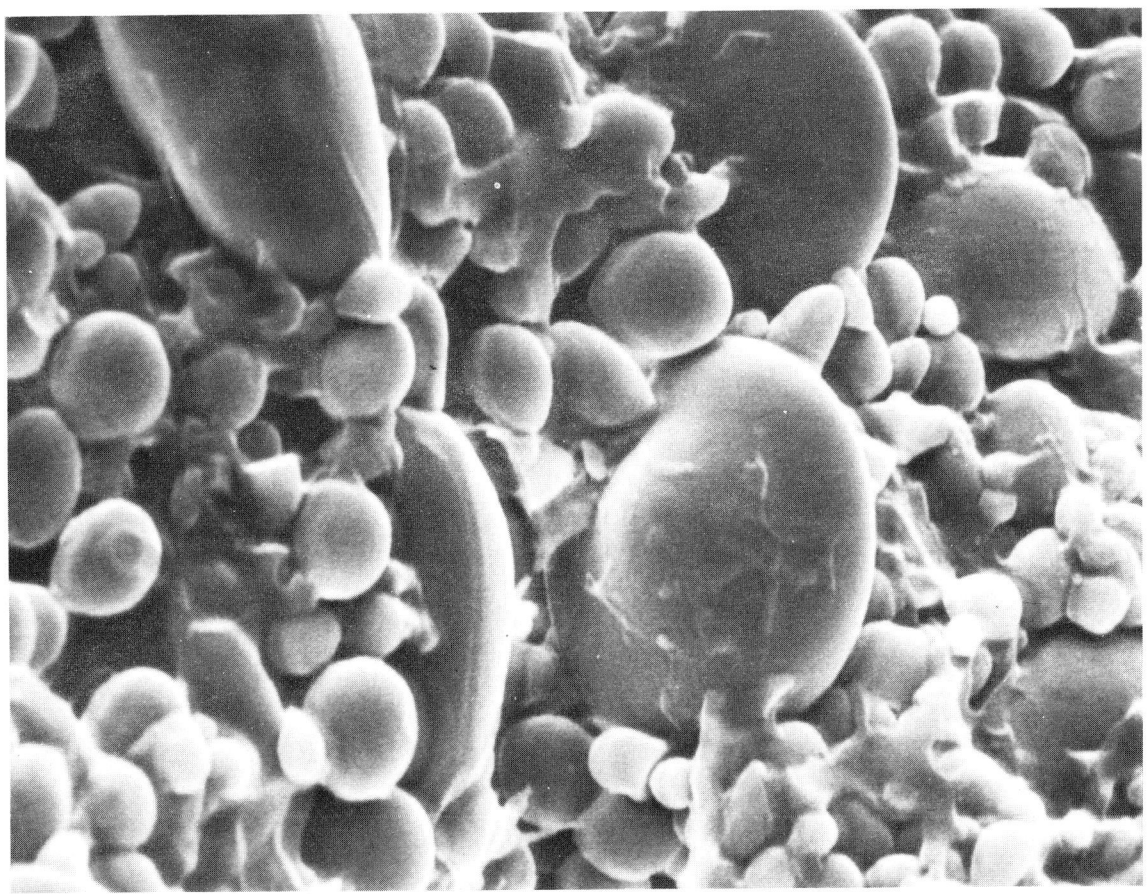

Starch granules raw.

maltose is composed of two glucose molecules. Next stage up from the simple single or double sugars comes *starch*, made up of numerous glucose units, linked together as a long chain, or *polysaccharide*. It is in this form that most plants store up the carbohydrates they have manufactured. Some, like the potato, store starch in their tubers; others, like the cassava, from which we get tapioca, have starch-rich roots. Seeds, such as those of the cereal crops, are also good sources of starch. Unripe fruits, too, are largely starch which is gradually converted to sugar as they ripen.

Starch is insoluble, but plants are able to convert it to soluble sugars when the occasion demands – and some of our digestive juices have the same facility. Looking at starchy foods under the microscope, however, shows that the starches come in the form of microscopic granules which vary from plant to plant, and around which there is an obvious 'skin'. Before our digestive juices can properly get at the starch to convert it into

Where do sugars come from?

Sugar	Source	Remarks
Glucose	Grapes and other fruits	
Liquid glucose	Maize starch	Used medically and in confectionery
Fructose	Fruit and honey	The sweetest of the sugars
Sucrose	Sugar cane, sugar beet	Household sugar, composed of fructose and glucose
Lactose	All kinds of milk	Less sweet than sucrose
Maltose	Germinating grains (malt)	Basis for fermentation in brewing

energy-giving glucose, the granules need to be broken up, and that is what happens in cooking.

The most complicated of carbohydrate structures is called cellulose and is built up of thousands of glucose units. This polysaccharide is the tough fibrous material found in wood and in the skin and frameworks of fruits, vegetables and cereals. The various celluloses are so complicated and securely locked together (in stiff parallel chains of sugars, rather than the spiral chains of starch molecules) that we cannot break them down in our bodies. They are useless as nutrients, but they do increase food's bulk and stimulate the movements of intestinal muscles. In a word, they provide *roughage*. It is now increasingly held that roughage, specifically from plant cellulose and particularly from the 'skin' or bran layers of wheat, plays a vital role not only in maintaining positive health and fitness but also in preventing a number of diseases. There is more on the bran scene in Chapter Six.

Again turning the microscope on plant tissue, it can be seen that those starch granules are themselves confined within cellulose frameworks. Cooking causes the starch granules to swell and gelatinise, thus giving them a soft texture and making them easier to digest.

Once the carbohydrates have been broken down into the simple single sugars – mainly glucose – they can be oxidised by body cells to produce energy and heat. Waste products from this process are carbon dioxide, which filters back through the bloodstream to be expelled through the lungs, and water.

Obviously, if we want 'instant' energy we should eat pure glucose, for it is quickly absorbed and ready for use. Sucrose, too, takes little time to be broken down, but as with any sugar it only

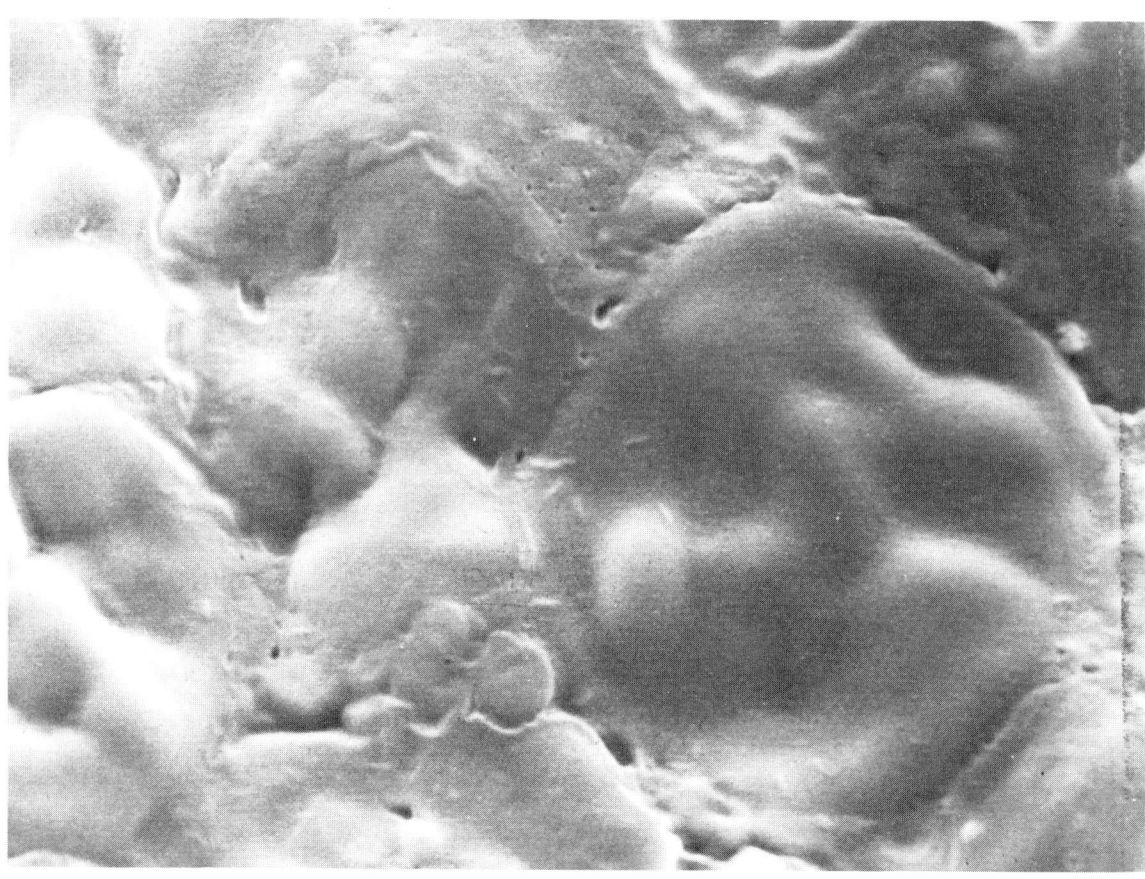

Starch granules after cooking: soft and gelatinous.

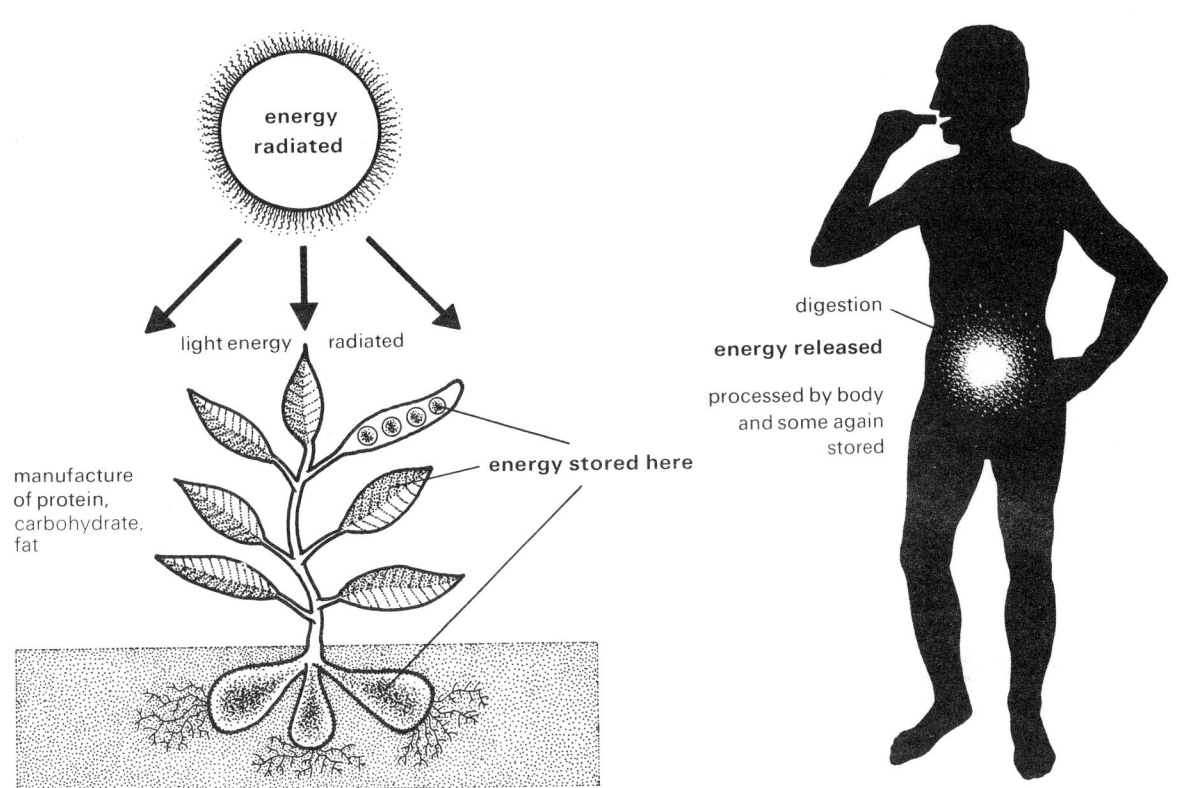

Solar energy is stored in plants: on being digested plants release their stored energy to the body.

supplies what the nutritionists call 'empty Calories' since it is purely an energy source and contains no protective, regulatory or body-building nutrients.

Both fructose and galactose, as well as glucose, are present in the bloodstream but since glucose is by far the commonest 'blood sugar' we will concentrate on what happens to that.

The *pancreas*, a gland at the back of the abdomen (we call it a *sweetbread* in animals) secretes a hormone called *insulin* which converts glucose into *glycogen*, sometimes called animal starch. Some of it is manufactured in muscle tissue, where it can be quickly broken down again when demands for action are made. Glycogen is also stored in the liver and in prolonged activity is re-processed to glucose to replenish muscular supplies.

But if we take in more glucose than we can use immediately or convert into glycogen, then the excess is processed into fat, which is simply an easier way of storing nutrients with energy-giving potential. Unfortunately too much of it is unsightly, it means that the body has to work harder carrying around all that extra weight, and obesity upsets body chemistry with potentially dangerous effects.

Fats: compact energy sources

Weight for weight, fats provide twice as many Calories as proteins or carbohydrates. They are also very satisfying and when food is in short supply as in, say, wartime rationing, fats are among the things people miss most.

Oils are the same sort of substances as fats, except that they are liquid at room temperature. In the heat of our stomachs the fats are melted down to oils.

Such substances contain a sweet, sticky liquid known as *glycerine* or *glycerol* (the same stuff used in fruit pastilles) combined chemically with an acid.

There are 25 different acids not illogically known as the '*fatty acids*', the commonest being *palmitic acid. stearic acid* and *oleic acid*. You may also come across *butyric acid*, found in butter (from which it gets its name), milk and cream.

Like the carbohydrates, the fats are made up of atoms of carbon, hydrogen and oxygen, but their proportions are different, with much less oxygen in the fats. Both plants and animals can make fats by chemical processes in which oxygen is removed from sugars, particularly glucose.

Different types of fat are produced by different types of fatty acid bonded with the glycerine. There are differences, too, in the make-up of the fatty acids, in particular in the number of hydrogen atoms within their complex molecular structure. Those that have the maximum number of hydrogen atoms are known as '*saturated*' fatty acids, while those linked together in a rather different way with fewer hydrogen atoms in their chemical chains are known as '*unsaturated*' fatty acids.

The saturated fats – that is, those formed by glycerol and a saturated fatty acid – are in general solid at room temperature. Beef and mutton fat, butter and lard are cardinal examples.

The unsaturated fats, which include most vegetable oils, such as olive, corn and sunflower oils, are usually liquid.

The role of fats in health and disease is the subject of much current controversy. The eating of the saturated varieties raises the levels of certain fatty substances in our blood called *cholesterol* and the *triglycerides*. Eating unsaturated fats can help to lower them. Cholesterol and the triglyceride levels seem to be related to the incidence of heart attacks, but just how directly they are linked remains a matter for heated medical debate. Many doctors, however, are convinced that by cutting down on animal fats – butter, milk, fatty meat, lard, dripping, eggs and

How much carbohydrate?

Carbohydrate Level	Type of Food	Examples:	% carbohydrate (weight)	Calories per oz
High 45–100% by weight	Cereal foods	Sweet biscuits	66	148
		Cake	60	variable
		Bread	50	66
		'Slimming rolls'	46	65
	Preserves etc.	Sugar	100	112
		Jam	70	74
		Chocolate	53	164
	Fruits	Dates	64	70
		Raisins	64	70
Medium 15–20% by weight	Fruit and vegetables	Grapes	15	20
		Bananas	20	22
		Potatoes	20	23 (boiled)
	Dairy Products	Milk	5	18
		Double Cream	2	128
		Butter	0	211
		Cheese	0	117
		Eggs	0	45
	Meat and Fish	Meat	0	60–90
		Fish	0	20–50
Low 0–10% by weight		Bacon	0	135
		Sausage	10	105
	Fruit and vegetables	Apples	10	13
		Oranges	10	7
		Plums	10	9
		Grapefruit	5	5
		Peas	10	14
		Sprouts	5	5
		Onions	5	7
		Cabbage	5	2
		Tomatoes	3	4
		Runner Beans	3	4
		Lettuce	2	3

Some of the fats

Name	Source	Remarks
Saturated fatty acids		
Butyric	Butter	Nutritional experts
Palmitic	suet and other	think these animal
Stearic	solid animal fats	fats may well
		contribute to
		heart disease if
		over-used
Unsaturated fatty acids		
Oleic	Olive oil	Nearly all of these
		are vegetable oils,
		and are considered
		more healthy.
Linoleic	Corn, soya,	These are called
	linseed	*Poly-unsaturated*,
Linolenic	Linseed	and are essential in
Arachidonic	Small amounts	the diet as the body
	in some animal	cannot make them
	fats	

so on – and concentrating on the vegetable fats, we could drastically lower the incidence of heart disease.

We will be looking in depth at diet and the coronary controversy in Chapter Five.

One fat fact that *is* certain is that animal fats, particularly those from butter, 'fat fish' like herring, salmon and sardine and from liver, naturally contain protective material in the form of vitamins A and D. These are not found in vegetable oils. Margarine, these days made largely from vegetable oils, has to have these vitamins added to give it the same protective value, as well as energy potential, as butter.

It is hard to define an absolute minimum daily fat intake level below which health is affected. The average adult in Britain takes in about 25 per cent of his total Calorie requirements in fat. It comes both in 'visible' fats, butter, margarine, cooking fats and oils and the like; and 'invisible' fats present in many other foods.

Fat is particularly useful to children, since it is a concentrated energy source. Youngsters have high energy requirements, as every parent knows, but small stomachs. The fats give concentrated energy without overloading the stomach.

The satisfying quality of the fats comes both from their lubricating properties – in cooking *and* eating – and because they are the most slowly digested nutrients.

When our fat intake is excess to requirements, the extra is stored. Although we obviously do not want too much extra to carry about – it is unsightly as well as unhealthy – we need at least a little fat insulation to help keep out the cold. Fat deposits are particularly useful in protecting some internal organs, notably the kidneys, which are vulnerable to cold.

It is fat deposits, too, which give women their characteristic shape – although Rubenesque rotundity seems now to have been replaced by angularity *à la* Twiggy.

Balancing the diet

The secret of healthy eating, of course, lies in taking in the proper proportions of all the nutrients. Excess proteins, it has been noted, can be used as energy providers; excess carbohydrates may be stored as fat. But if any of the different food factors is missing, the body will not remain in tip-top condition.

Carbohydrates, for example, are desirable (in moderation) because they are 'protein sparers': unless protein and carbohydrate are eaten together, the valuable amino-acids will be burned for energy instead of being used for body-cell building and repair. Good examples of protein/carbohydrate mixtures are the traditional British fish and chips, bread and cheese, meat and potatoes.

It is also important that fats and carbohydrates are taken together, otherwise the fats are incompletely burned up, forming rather nasty waste products which cause sickness and headaches and a loss of appetite. An example of a good carbohydrate/fat combination is bread and butter. Cakes, too, nicely combine fats and carbohydrates.

In Britain we eat carbohydrates, proteins and fats in a rough proportion of 4:1:1. In many other parts of the world the carbohydrates, usually in the form of cereals (made into bread) or rice, form a much bigger part of the diet. It is usually recommended that they should never exceed two-thirds of the total energy intake, but they frequently do.

There are many difficulties in obtaining a balanced diet. First, there is sheer availability, not a problem in the still relatively affluent West, but a pressing concern over much of the globe.

Then, of course, there is the problem that you cannot tell simply by looking at foods how much of the various factors they have in them. That

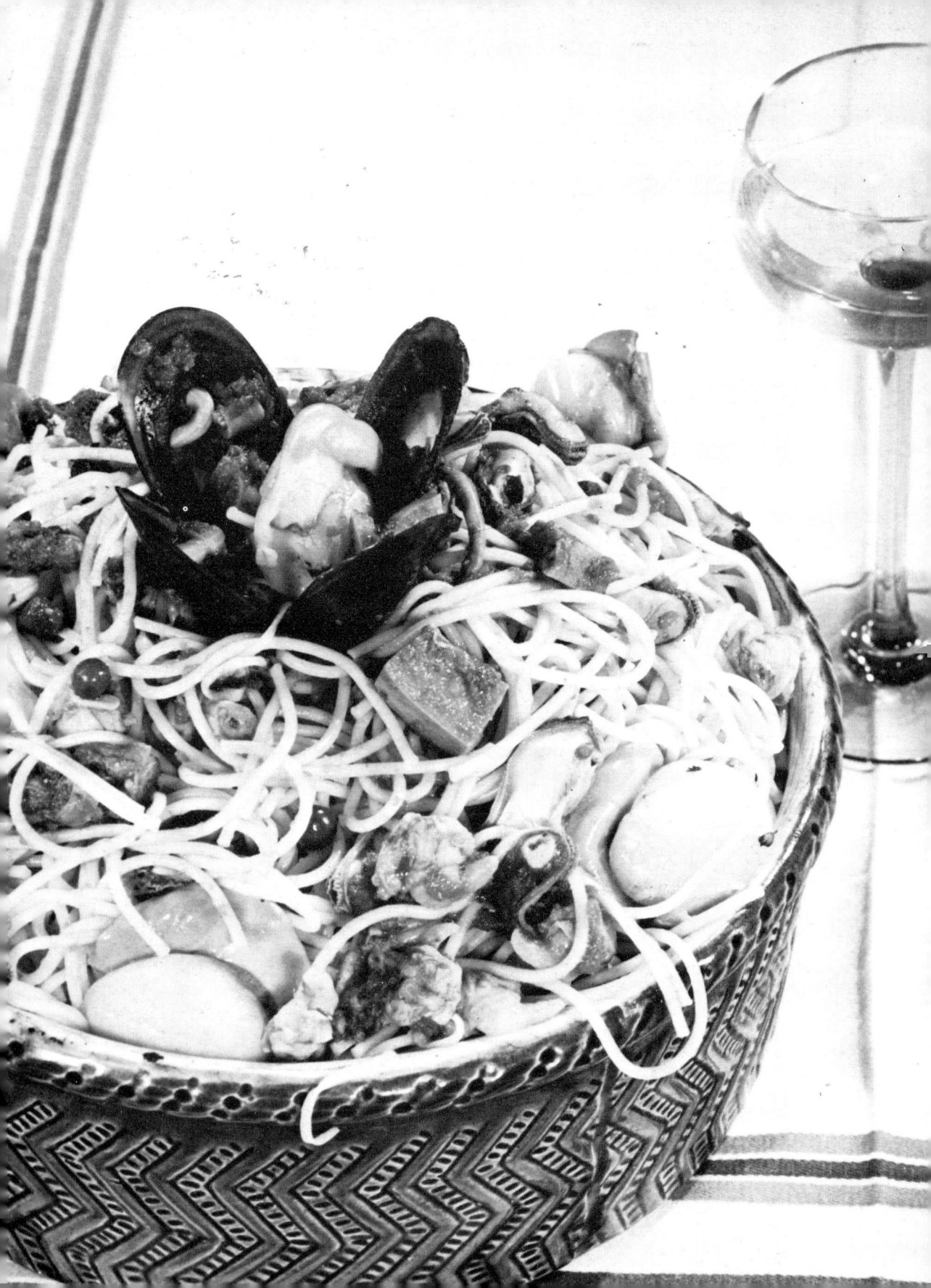

takes knowledge and experience and many of us, I am afraid, are woefully nutritionally ill-educated.

And lastly there is that terrible perversion of 'hunger', by 'appetite'.

All these factors have led to an extraordinarily wide variety in the kind of food we eat. Despite this world–wide variety, however, there are those who claim that only certain foods grown in a certain way, and uncontaminated with certain additives are 'natural' for man to eat. But is there such a thing as a natural food? Which additives are permissible and which are not? This is the subject of the next chapter.

What is a balanced meal? Examples from N. Europe, the Mediterranean and Asia.

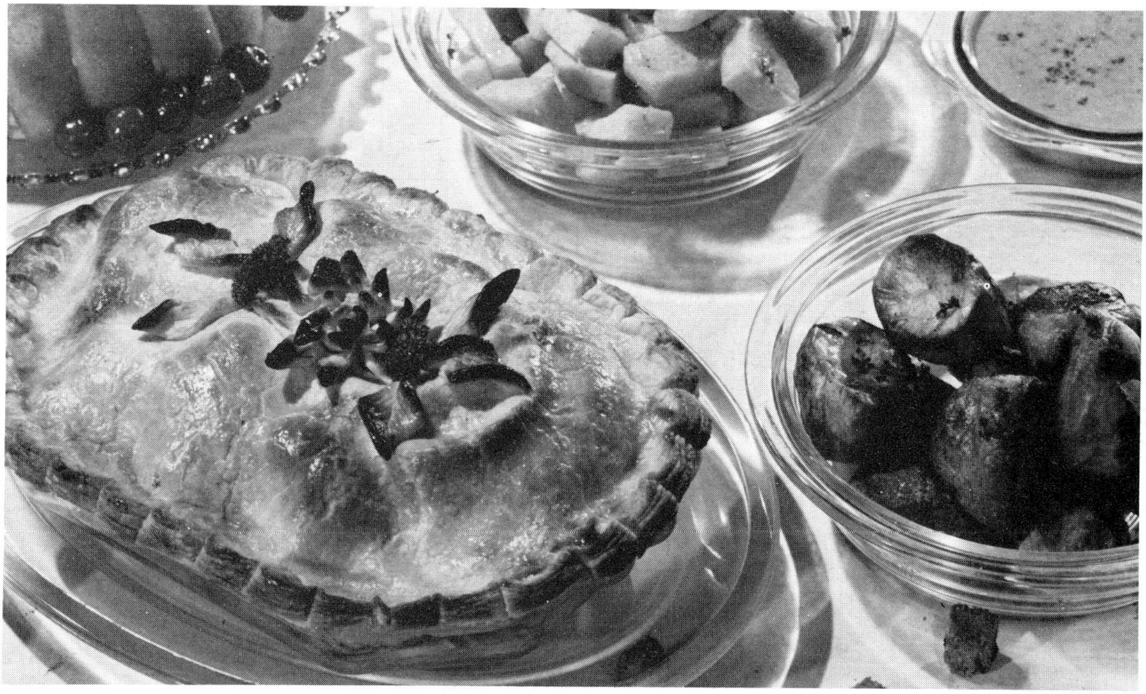

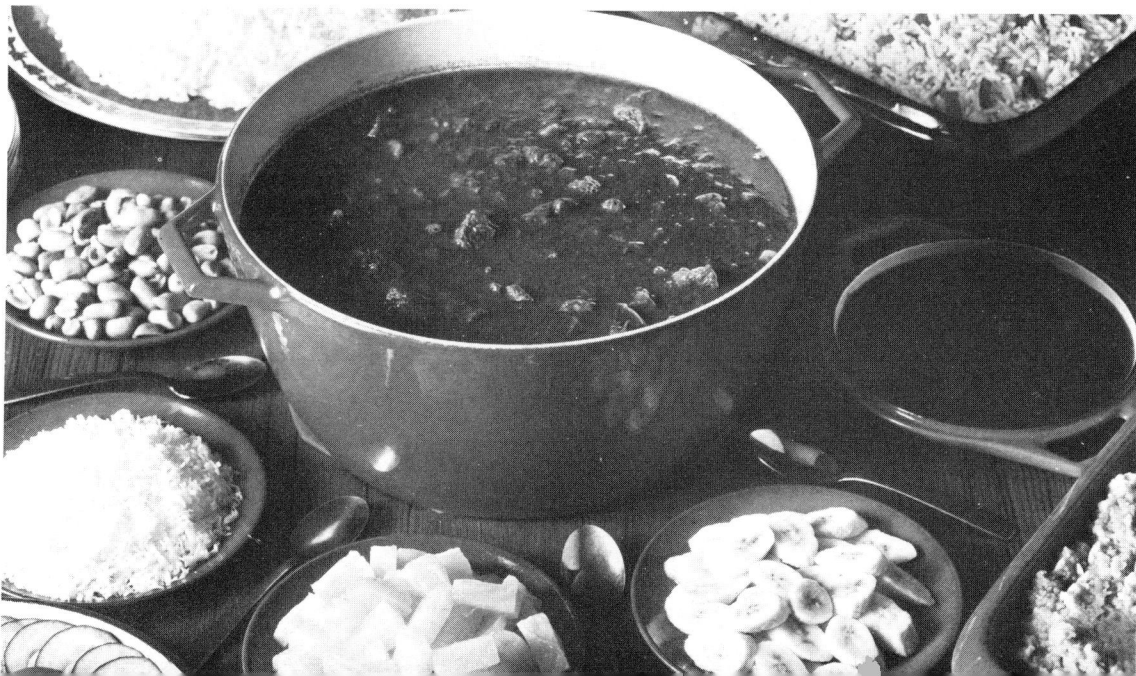

3 How natural is natural? Additives

'Their best and most wholesome feeding is upon one dish and no more, and the same plain and simple: for surely this huddling of many meats one upon another of diverse tastes is pestiferous. But sundry sauces are more dangerous than that.'

Pliny, Historia Naturalis, Book Nine.

'Many dishes make many diseases.'

Thomas Moffett, 'Health's Improvement'.

'Last year each of us, on average, swallowed three pounds of flavourings, colouring, preservatives, glazes, anti-spattering agents, emulsifiers, bleaches and other additives with our food.'

Dr Joan Morgan in 'Medical News'.

'Vegetable protein, onion, cornflour, leek, tomato, carrot, salt, beef fat, edible starch, guar gum, autolysed yeast, hydrolysed protein, monosodium glutamate, wheatflour, tricalcium phosphate, sugar, caramel, ascorbic acid, flavour, emulsifier, nicotinic acid, reduced iron, antioxidant, retinyl palmitate, thiamine hydrochloride, riboflavin and cholecalciferol.'

List of ingredients on a packet of 'beef-flavour casserole'.

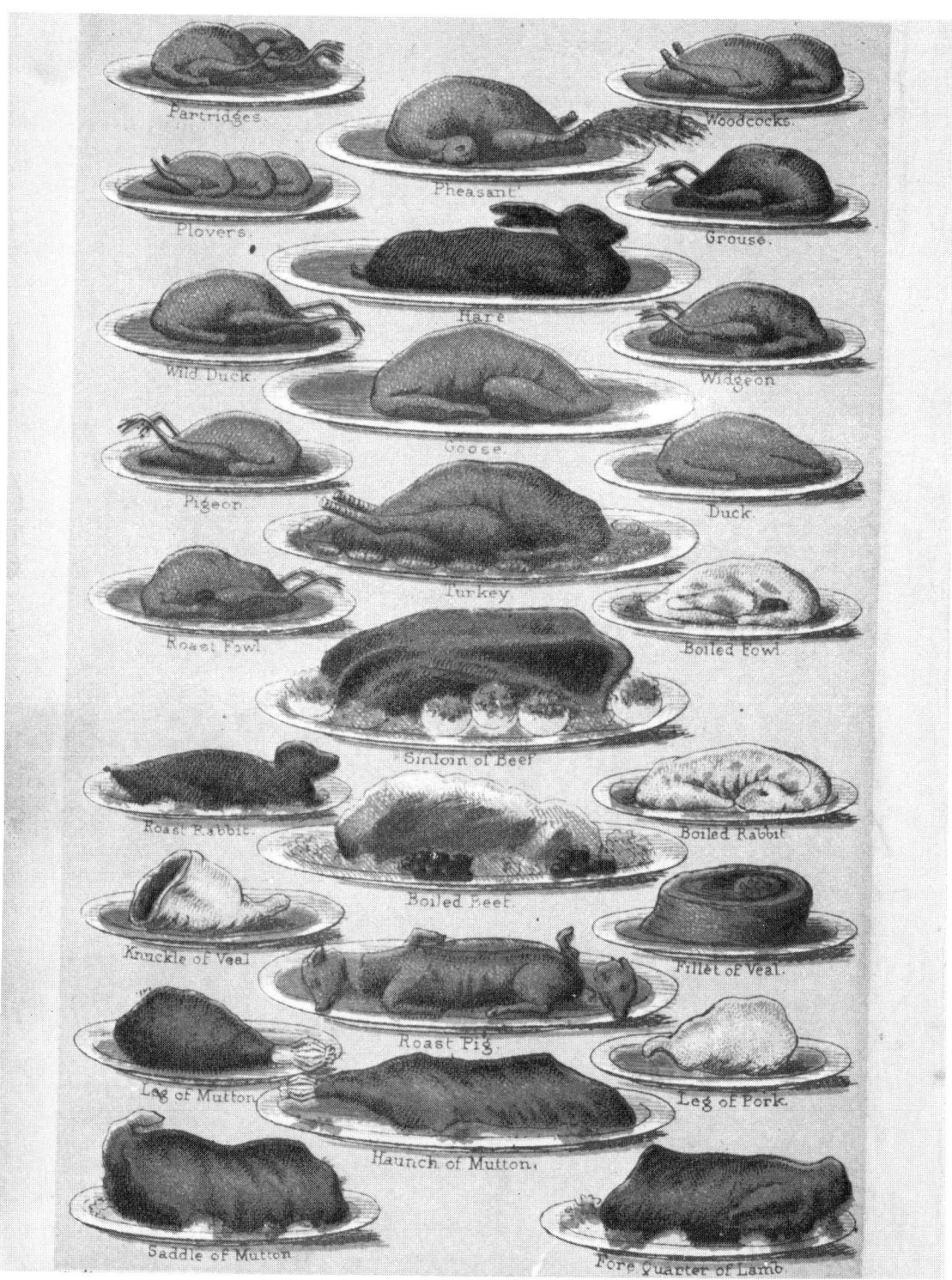

Glories of Victorian cooking.

I have always like the story of the man in the restaurant who asked the waiter what he would recommend. 'The tongue's very good, sir,' came the reply. 'The tongue!' said the man. 'You don't expect me to eat something that's come out of an animal's mouth, do you? . . Bring me an egg!'

More than likely the tale is apocryphal but it does demonstrate the complete lack of logic applied to defining which foods are 'natural' or reasonable to eat. In the first chapter we saw the wide variety of ways in which man chooses to take in his food. A Frenchman won't eat dog, as the Polynesians do, but seems happy enough with horse. We may shudder as he dangles a snail on his forchette but wonder why our Jewish orthodox cousins abhor the flesh of the pig.

And what is intrinsically the matter with deep-fried termite, roast grasshopper in soy sauce or canned wasp maggot, those sought-after Eastern delicacies?

Like it or not man is an omnivore and takes his nourishment where he may. There is no such thing as natural food and what we eat is dictated by tradition and habit, taboo and history.

Yet these days you will hear much about 'natural foods', especially from those who believe that 'they' (whoever 'they' may be) are slowly poisoning us all, sapping our vitality and our

virility by feeding us nasty synthetic foods, full of noxious chemical additives. Further, many of them believe that so-called natural foods untainted by 'chemicals' (although all food, as we have seen, is composed of chemicals) have positive benefits, additional properties which revive and stimulate. For example, as Magnus Pyke has pointed out: 'A significant number of people believe that foods manured with dung possess special virtues other than those measurable by scientific observation.'

Now there is no denying that if you feel something is doing you good, it usually *will* do you good, and doctors and medical research workers are paying increasing attention to this psychosomatic effect.

Apart from that, however, can we show that 'natural foods' are superior, or that synthetic foods are insidiously poisoning us? In Chapter Four food processing techniques will be discussed in detail. Here the spotlight is on food *additives*, both using so-called natural products and synthetic ones.

The practice of adding chemicals to food, particularly to preserve it, has been carried on for millennia. Salting and pickling are obvious examples, but they have been going on so long that we regard the foods so produced as entirely 'natural'. Similarly colouring and flavouring agents have long been in use. The argument in

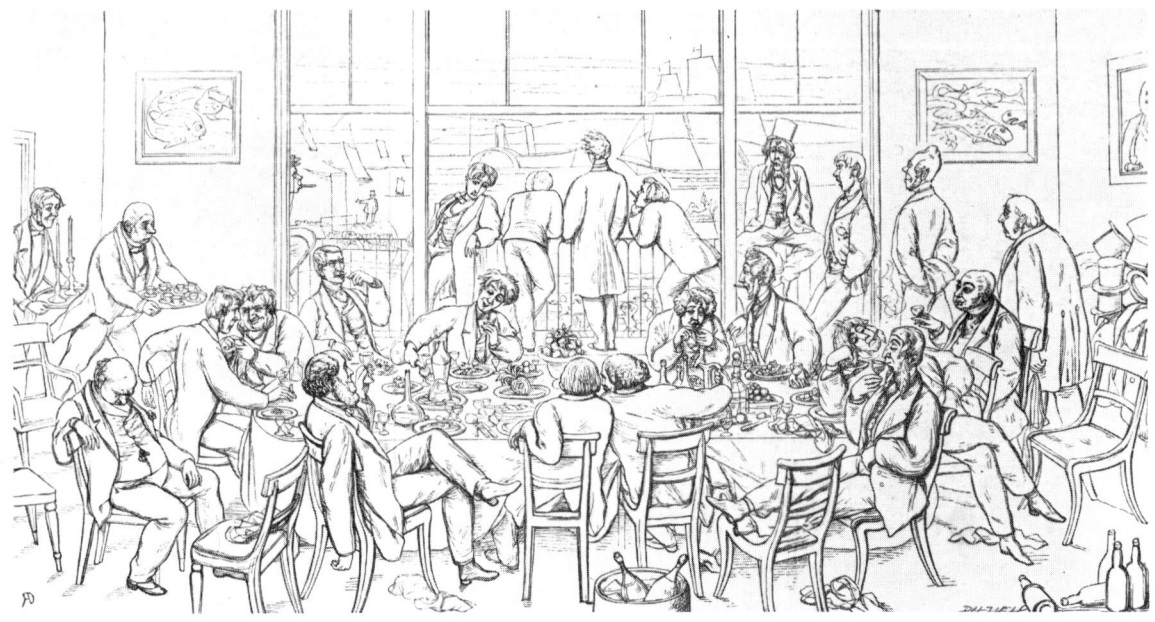

Overdoing it at table, 19th Century style.

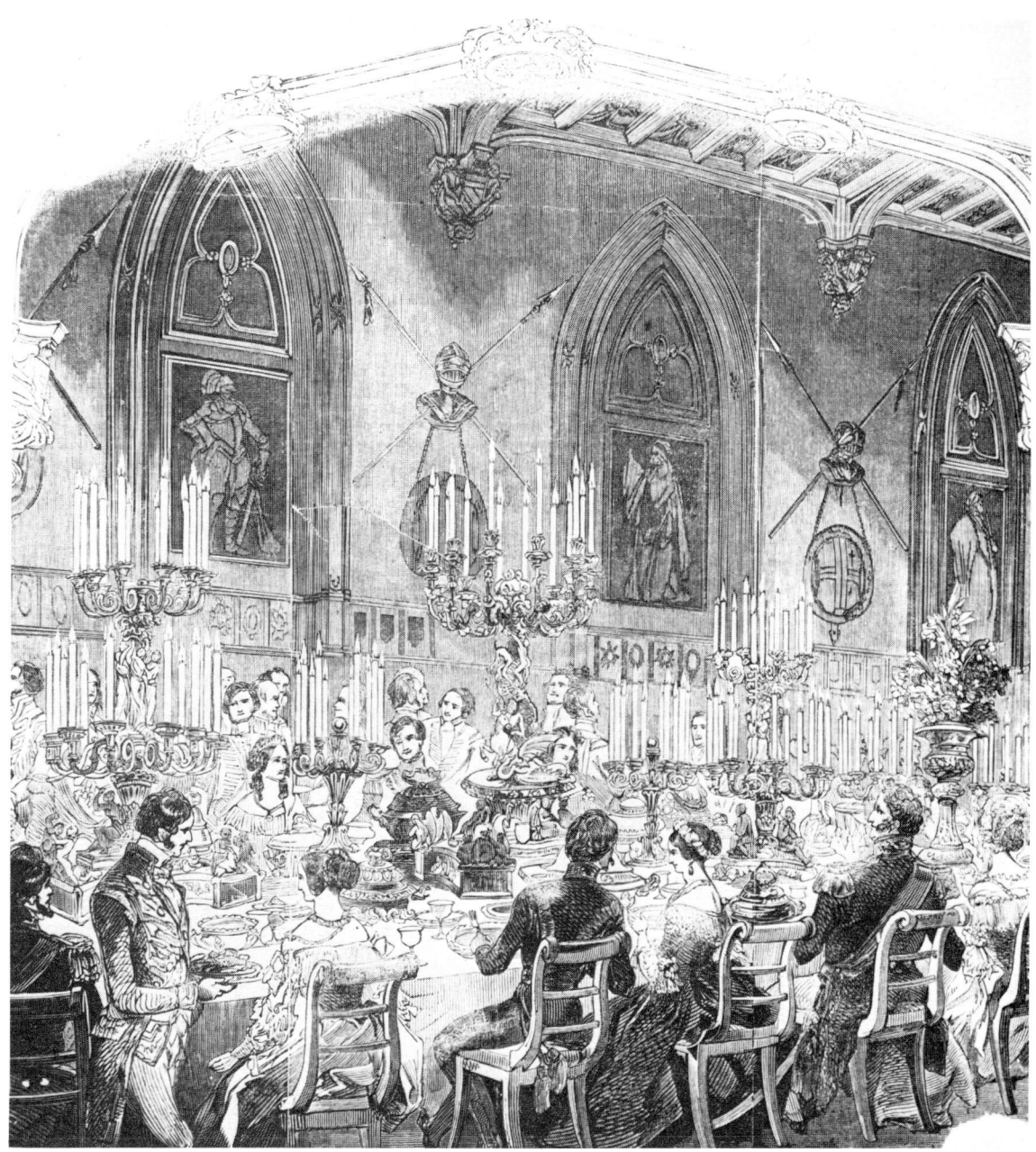

The opulence of Victorian banquets.

favour of such products, however, is that they must be safe since they have been used for so long without killing anyone. But is that really true? When we apply to the old additives the rigorous testing criteria we use for the new ones – something, incidentally, done most infrequently – we can uncover some disturbing facts. For instance, a 'natural' substance called *safrole*, obtained from the bark of the sassafras tree, had been flavouring American root beer for many years. Stringent testing showed that it can produce liver cancer in rats, and its use was prohibited.

But it is not just additives that may bring dangers. Many natural products themselves contain potentially-deadly poisons, although they only occasionally seem to do their consumers much harm. Nonetheless, were we to have applied today's food testing standards to, say, the potato, it would never have been passed for human consumption.

How safe is the potato?

Potatoes contain a highly-toxic substance called *solanine*. It is normally present in very small quantities of around 90 to 100 parts per million, but the concentration increases rapidly if the potatoes are left in the sun and allowed to turn green and at concentrations of 400 parts per

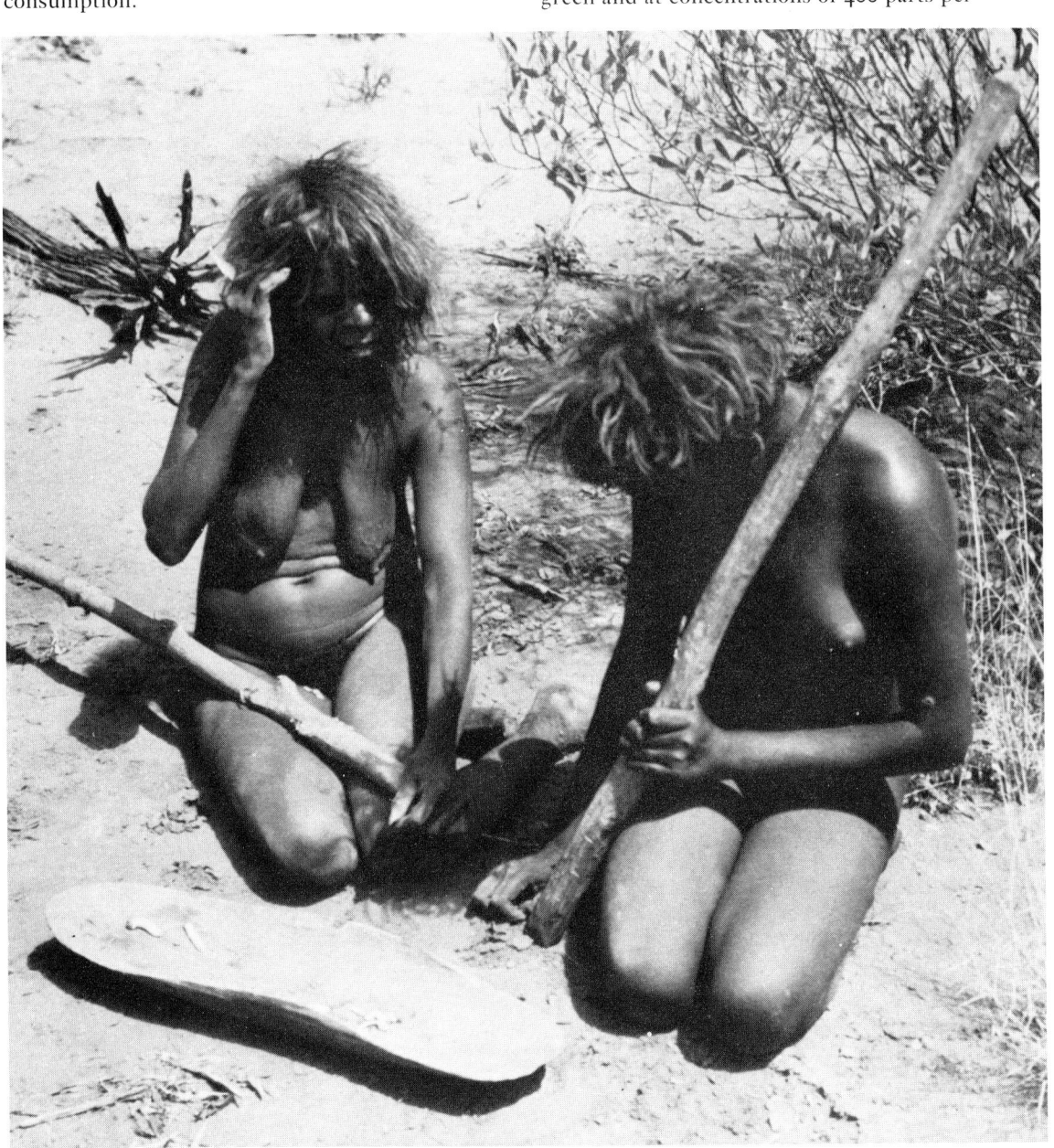

Australian nomads include nutritious grubs in their diet.

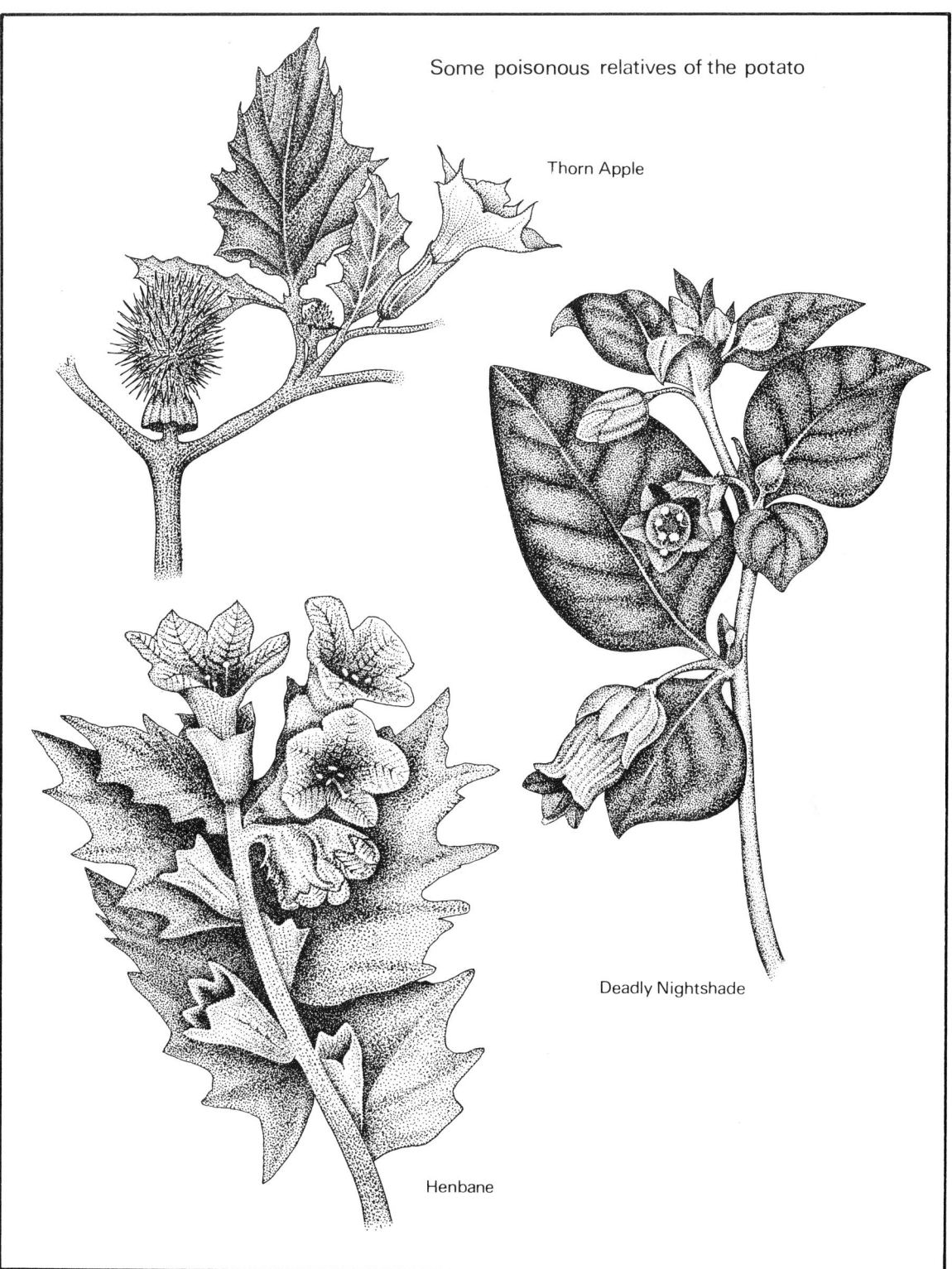

Some poisonous relatives of the potato

Thorn Apple

Deadly Nightshade

Henbane

million or so, serious food poisoning can result. The reason why we are seldom disturbed by the potatoes we eat is that most solanine is concentrated in the green patches which are usually cut out before cooking. Boiling, too, extracts some of the poison.

As far as artificial products and additives are concerned, however, it is normal to insist on a safety factor of 100. That is, the maximum amounts allowed are usually one-hundredth of the amount known to cause toxic effects in animals. When the foods in question are commonly eaten by children the safety factor may be increased to 150 or even 200.

Yet we seem happily to eat potatoes which, before cooking and preparation at least, can contain toxic solanine at a concentration of only one quarter or a fifth of levels known to cause poisoning in humans, let alone experimental animals.

It is interesting also to note the progress of one current theory that blighted potatoes could be the cause of that distressing congenital birth complaint, spina bifida. Dr J. H. Renwick of London School of Hygiene and Tropical Medicine had apparently established a link between the incidence of the disease and the fluctuating occurrence of potato blight, especially in countries with high potato consumption, like Ireland. His hypothesis was supported by the work of Professor D. E. Poswillo, Professor of Teratology at the Royal College of Surgeons, who fed potato blight extracts to marmosets during pregnancy. Many of the fetuses developed severe defects.

Subsequent work, mainly of a statistical and epidemiological nature has, happily, failed to confirm any link between spina bifida and potato blight. But public, parliamentary and governmental reaction to the early findings of Renwick and Poswillo was subdued, in sharp contrast, for example, to the brouhaha over cyclamates and their subsequent banning. Now grave doubts have been cast on the evidence suggesting that cyclamates are harmful. Why did we act so stridently and, it seems, precipitously, over a synthetic product yet appear so little concerned over a natural one?

I'm strong to the finish 'cos I eats my spinach

We may not actively encourage our children to eat potatoes but few parents, I suspect, would hesitate to recommend the virtues of rhubarb and, thanks to Popeye, spinach. Yet the leaves of both contain *oxalic acid*, a substance toxic to both man and animals since it combines with and 'captures' calcium, thus severely diminishing the levels of that vital mineral in the bloodstream. A study of some sheep which died after eating rhubarb leaves, for example, showed blood calcium levels were one-fifth of normal. This led, among other symptoms, to reduced coagulability, acute inflammation of the kidney and disturbances of the nervous system.

A talented family

The Nightshades (Solanaceae)	By-products
Edible	
Potato (tubers only)	
Tomato	
Sweet Pepper	fruit only
Aubergine	
Chili	
Capsicum	
Tobacco (smoking and chewing)	Nicotine, *extremely* poisonous in quantity. Used against insects
Very poisonous	
Belladonna (deadly nightshade)	Atropine, used in medicine
Bittersweet	
Woody Nightshade	
Henbane	Hyoscine, used for travel sickness
Thorn apple	
Ornamental	
Nicotiana	
Petunia	

How to eat nettles

Young nettles are a pleasant vegetable something like spinach. But they do not contain oxalic acid as spinach does. They must be picked when young and pale green (with gloves!), as the older ones are tough and stringy. You need a large saucepan full to provide a helping, as they boil down like spinach. Bring about 1 cupful of water to a brisk boil, throw in the freshly picked and cut-up nettles and a pinch of salt. Cook rapidly until ready (usually about 4 minutes).

In laboratory experiments, animals were fed spinach in conjunction with a low calcium diet: it proved fatal.

Now, by and large, people do not eat large enough quantities of these vegetables (rhubarb is technically a vegetable although it usually masquerades as a fruit) for the oxalic acid content to do any apparent harm. And as far as rhubarb is concerned, most of the acid is concentrated in the leaves. Even so, lower concentrations can in certain circumstances, be harmful. During the food shortages of the First World War, people were officially recommended to eat rhubarb leaves, and several were fatally poisoned. There is a case on record in America of a woman dying within 36 hours of a meal of fried rhubarb leaves.

Of cabbages and kale. . .

Iodine, as we have seen (chapter one, p.27) is vital for the production of the hormone *thyroxine*. Lack of iodine leads to an unsightly swelling of the thyroid gland in the neck, called a goitre. Such swelling can also cause undue pressure on neighbouring structures, such as the windpipe, veins and nerves. In areas where the soil lacks iodine, goitre is endemic. There used, for example, to be a 'goitre belt' running from Derbyshire through to Somerset. Indeed, 'Derbyshire Neck' is another name for the condition.

Goitre has been largely overcome, in most parts of the world by adding traces of iodine to table salt. In Tasmania, however, it was found in 1955 that the incidence of the condition was increasing, despite the use of iodised salt. It was discovered that, in order to increase their milk yield, farmers had been switching to a new feed, called 'many headed kale'. This contains a substance known as *oxazolidine* which prevents the accumulation of sufficient quantities of iodine in the thyroid, even when there is enough of it in the diet. The cows were getting it from the kale and passing it on to the children in their contaminated milk.

Nearly 30 years earlier researchers in America had noticed a number of laboratory rats, fed mainly on cabbage, developed goitre and follow-up investigations in New Zealand inculpated turnips too. Mustard seed and rape seed were also found to contain oxazolidine.

In fact, quite a number of green vegetables – brussels sprouts, broccoli and kohlrabi, as well as cabbage, kale and turnips – contain this goitre-producing substance.

Of course, when iodine supplies are more than adequate the tiny amounts of oxazolidine that we actually take in have little or no physiological effect. Nonetheless, as the Tasmanian experience showed, natural products can even at second hand have undesirable side-effects.

The cup that cheers?

And what about those entirely natural, non-alcoholic beverages, tea and coffee, inbibed by most of us all at regular intervals throughout the day. Each cup contains about 0·05 to 0·1 grams of that stimulant drug caffeine, 10 grams of which can be a fatal dose in humans? It is true that we are unlikely to swallow 100 to 200 cups a day, but the rats who developed cancer when fed cyclamates were given that substance in amounts which were equivalent to an 11-stone man drinking *500 8oz bottles of cyclamate-sweetened soft drinks for every day of his life*! Those rats fed the equivalent of *200 bottles a day* did not develop tumours.

Nobody would seriously suggest banning tea, coffee, cabbage, rhubarb and spinach from the

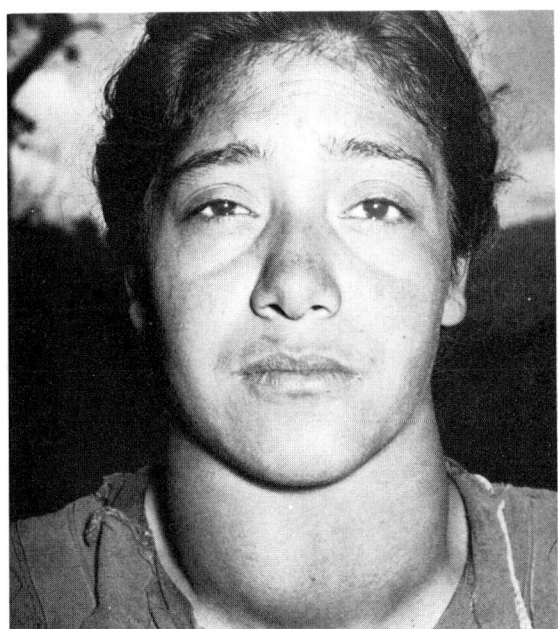

Goitre.

D

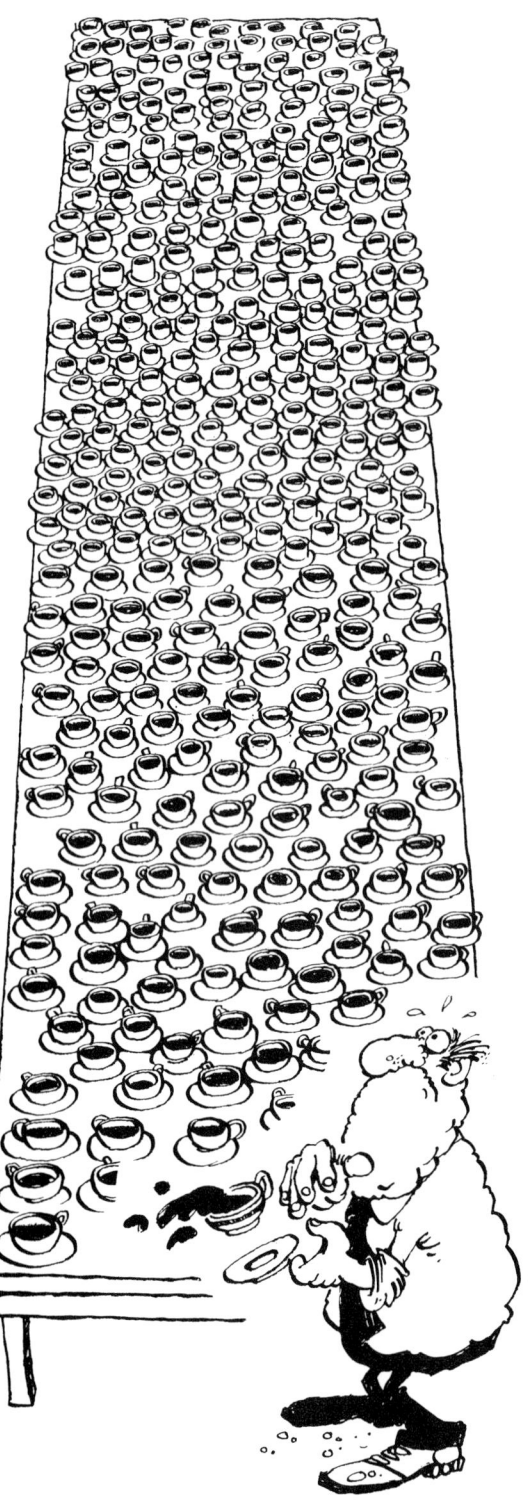

"True, we are unlikely to swallow 100 cups a day . . ."

nation's diet. We have, after all, been eating and drinking them for generations. They have stood their test, that of time. But what about avocados? Quoting from Magnus Pyke's *Food and Society*: 'Avocados . . . are a delicacy. By what right or logic, therefore, have they escaped pharmacological scrutiny? Not only have instances of poisoning been reported among cattle, horses, goats, rabbits, canaries and fish after having eaten them, but when they were submitted to test in the laboratory, the fruit and the leaves as well were found to contain a toxic substance.

'The effect on animals may be serious. Cows, goats and mares develop acute mastitis. Goats may be so severely poisoned that they die. . . A curious case reported by Professor Kingsbury was that of canaries fed on ripe avocado pears being poisoned.

'Although avocados do not as a general rule form a major part of human diets, nevertheless it is perhaps paradoxical that such an exotic food should have escaped scrutiny by nutritionists although the canary, used as a sensitive detector of air unfit for men in coal-mines and submarines, has proved to be susceptible also to this new danger.'

To this list of potentially-hazardous natural products should be added the onion which in animals, notably dogs and horses, can cause anaemia; a certain variety of broad bean, *Vicia fava*, which can precipitate a disease, favism, characterised by diarrhoea and anaemia; and horseradish, the roots of which have killed cattle, horses and pigs.

The safety margins, as regards the onion, do not seem that high. Extrapolating the dog experiment, it seems one would have regularly to eat about three-quarters of a pound of onions a day to bring on anaemia. That level of consumption seems a far more likely possibility than those hundreds of bottles of cyclamate sweetened soft drinks.

Although the onion certainly adds savour to our diets, it is not very important nutritionally. Recent evidence, however, suggests that onions, and to a greater extent, garlic, might be important in reducing the incidence of coronary thrombosis. (In one experiment at the University of Newcastle's Department of Medicine, 22 patients were given a fried, fatty breakfast and, as expected, this adversely affected the biochemical factors associated with blood clotting.

On other days, when the same patients were given the same breakfasts, but with an additional two-ounce portion of onions, there was a significant decrease in the 'blood clotting parameters'. Researchers in several centres are at present trying to isolate the active ingredient from onions and garlic cloves.)

For most people the broad bean brings positive nutritional benefits: those who contract favism do so because of a genetically-determined defect, the lack of a particular enzyme in their blood. If favism were caused by a synthetic nutrient would we ban its use in the whole population because of the inherited susceptibility of a minority?

From time to time we hear of certain foods being implicated as possible causes of cancer. It has been firmly established, for example, that groundnuts can become contaminated with a poison, called *aflatoxin*, produced by a fungus which can grow on them. Turkeys, ducklings, pheasants, pigs, cattle have all been poisoned by this substance and laboratory tests show it to be one of the most active substances in producing malignant tumours in rats (although mice are unaffected). There is now strong circumstantial evidence that aflatoxin is involved in the high prevalence of certain human liver cancers in parts of Asia and Africa where groundnuts form an important part of the diet.

Steering a rational course

All these examples of potential dangers in natural foods are not intended as 'scare stories', to fill you with concern about every item of your diet. All they are intended to do is to demonstrate that absolute safety is impossible, that applying modern techniques we can find dangerous substances in the apparently most innocuous of foods.

Nor should they be taken as arguing that 'two wrongs make a right'. Just because we can identify toxins in natural products doesn't mean we should not exercise the greatest care in ensuring that they are not present in dangerous quantities in those substances which we are going deliberately to add to our diets.

They do, however, serve to demonstrate that the greatest care must be taken in interpreting the results of toxicity testing. Unfortunately such care is often not exercised, either by the media, or by some scientists who ought to know better.

It is seldom realised, or publicised, for example, that the aim of toxicity testing is to *produce* a toxic effect. What is important is the level of concentration at which animals *are* affected. Finding this level, in say microgrammes per kilogramme of body weight in various animals and then dividing by 100 or so – the safety factor – should give you safe levels.

One of America's problems in this field is the Delaney Amendment, an addition to the food and drugs laws which insists that if any substance is shown to cause cancer in experimental animals, *regardless of how high the dosage*, it has to be banned.

At the time of the cyclamates ban in the USA, the late Professor Alan Keckwick, chairman of Britain's food additives advisory committee, told me: 'This ruling could equally apply to sugar itself, canned meat and bacon. All these in massive doses can cause cancer in animals. Are we going to ban them?' The answer, of course, was no.

Allan Cameron in his book *Food – Facts and Fallacies* also makes a telling point: 'We may test our own reaction to the use of food additives by taking salt as an example. Salt is a pure chemical substance and in some recent experiments rats were fed salt at a level equivalent in man to one half to one ounce per day. The result was that the rats suffered from high blood pressure and died earlier than control rats fed on an ordinary diet. When the amount of salt was doubled they died still earlier, at an age equivalent to 32 in man.

'If we react the same way to the results of this experiment as several authorities did to the results of cyclamate experiments on rats, we would demand the banning of salt. Needless to say we do not react in this way at all: we regard salt as safe because it has been used for many centuries and we persuade ourselves that it is a natural and therefore above suspicion.' Before turning to modern additives let us look at the extraordinary range of traditional 'extras' our foods have contained for generations.

Some old-fashioned additives: preservation

Salt is as a food additive, with two distinct uses: in smallish doses, as a flavouring (and how tasteless food seems without salt) and in larger quantities, as a preservative.

Until comparatively recently, *the* method of preserving meat was to salt it, either by rubbing with dry salt or by pickling in brine. Salt, in common with other natural preservatives like sugar and vinegar, acts by killing off micro-organisms and inhibiting the action of enzymes which are necessary for the process of decay.

Today, the only form of meat salted on a very large scale is pork: the sides of the pig form bacon and the hind legs, hams. Although the old-fashioned way to produce these products is to rub dry salt into the pork, it is commoner nowadays to produce 'mild cured' ham and bacon by soaking in brine. They do not, however, keep as long as the dry-salted varieties. As well as killing micro-organisms in the meat, salt also partially dries it by extracting water from the tissues. Preservation time is further lengthened by smoking – hanging in the smoke from the sawdusts of hardwoods like oak or beech. Products in the smoke also have an antiseptic effect. With today's deep freezers and domestic refrigerators we salt and smoke bacon and ham for their flavour rather than their preservative properties.

Fish are frequently preserved by salting and some by smoking too, as in kippers, bloaters, Finnon Haddock and smoked salmon. Vegetables, notably beans, may also be preserved by storing them between layers of salt. The salt which is added to butter, cheese and margarine, while primarily there as a flavouring, does act as a preservative as well.

Sugar, too, has long been used as a food additive and in many products its fundamental role is one of preservation rather than taste-enhancement. Fruits are preserved by sugar as

Some hints on preserving food

Q *Why does food go bad?*

A Mostly because bacteria and molds grow in it, and convert it into unpalatable waste products.

Examples: *Milk* goes sour because *bacteria* digest the milk sugar into lactic acid. The acid then clots the protein the milk. BUT this isn't all bad – you can get:

Yoghourt
Curd cheese
Soured cream etc.

Stewed fruit goes fizzy because *yeasts* digest the sugar into alcohol and carbon dioxide. BUT properly controlled, this also gives WINE.

Meat stinks because bacteria and enzymes digest the protein. Not much benefit from this, unless you like your game slightly 'high'. The activities of these bacteria and enzymes can 'tenderise' tougher meats if kept in check.

Q *How can I prevent food from 'going off'?*

A There are four main methods of foiling microbes:

1 Heat

Nearly all bacteria, yeasts etc. are killed by boiling. So if you boil and then seal food in a container, it will stay unspoiled for some months, e.g. *Bottling* and *Canning.*

Warning: If the heating has not been thorough, some bacteria may remain, and can grow in sealed containers causing dangerous poisons to build up.

2 Pickling

A strong solution of *Salt* or of *Sugar* or of *Vinegar* acts as a deterrent for microbes.

e.g. Salted herrings
Salt beef
Jams and Jellies

Pickles (all three combined)

3 Smoking

This acts partly by drying – microbes are unhappy in a dry environment – and partly through the chemical action of substances in woodsmoke.

e.g. Ham
Kippers
Smoked Salmon

Drying on its own is often used for:

Apple rings
Herbs
Pemmican (the explorer's standby: strips of dried meat)

4 Cooling

Microbes need warmth in order to grow and multiply. An ordinary refrigerator simply keeps food at a *fairly* low temperature and allows us to keep it longer than in a warm kitchen.

A *freezer* actually takes it below freezing point and will preserve it for a very long time **as long as it is not allowed to thaw for any length of time.** Each time it warms up, bacteria get a chance to grow and multiply.

Microbes are not killed by cold, they only hibernate.

Q *If I keep food covered, won't that keep microbes out?*

A Definitely not. Bacteria and yeasts are everywhere, including on our skin, and you cannot reasonably expect to keep them out of food in ordinary home conditions. It is best not to keep food for long, unless you are confident you have used one of the methods shown above.

jams, jellies, marmalades or candied, glacé and crystallised fruits. High concentrations of sugar in and around the fruit inhibit the growth of moulds and yeasts. Some experts have questioned whether sugar in jam can be regarded as an additive since it is *the* main ingredient and you cannot make jam without it. But since the object surely is to preserve the fruit, rather than flavour the sugar, it must be the sugar rather than the fruit which is the additive. As a flavouring sugar finds its way into an extraordinarily large range of products: check your groceries next week and see how often it appears on the list of contents. In fact half of our daily sugar intake comes indirectly through eating other foods. The consequences of our enormous sugar consumption are discussed in detail in Chapter Five.

The other traditional preservative is vinegar, the active ingredient of which, *acetic acid*, stops spoilage by preventing the multiplication of micro-organisms. Vegetables are almost exclusively the foods that come in for the vinegar 'pickling' process, although a notable exception is the walnut. Salt and spices are usually added to the solution to give piquancy.

Chutneys, of fruit as well as vegetables, use all three of the traditional preserving additives: salt, sugar and vinegar.

More traditional additives: flavour and colouring

As we have seen in Chapter One, man has created an enormous variety of dishes to tickle his palate, and from time immemorial he has been adding substances to the animal and plant life he eats to enhance both their flavour and appearance. Although most of these additives have little or no food value in the strictly nutritional sense, they do play a significant role in our diets. For the 'taste' of food – and that includes colour and aroma as well as the straightforward excitement of the taste buds – is of great importance in stimulating the appetite and encouraging the flow of digestive juices.

And a few centuries ago certain additives, that is the spices, were absolutely essential if food was to be edible at all. Most animals were slaughtered before winter set in and the meat preserved by salting. By the end of the winter, however, it was usually very tough and often, despite the salt, had become 'high', mouldy and maggoty. Spices and herbs were essential to mask the repulsive flavour of tainted meat and to overcome the salty monotony. Even in Victorian times spices were among the grocer's most important commodities – a fact recognised still in the French name for the trade: *L'épicier*, the spicer.

Man's craving for spice was such that for many centuries world politics were dominated by their trade: Venice, for example, owes its glory to the purveying of spice. Vasco da Gama and Columbus had behind their explorations the stimulus of finding new routes to the spice islands of the East Indies. There are five main spice types, named after the part of the plant from which they originate: fruit, seed, flower, bark or root. Their efficacy is largely due to the so-called 'essential oils' they contain. Such oils are usually colourless and highly-volatile, with powerful smells and tastes.

Of the fruit spices, pepper is the most important. Black peppers are the unripe berries of a tropical creeping plant; white peppers are the same berries, picked when a little riper and with the outside skin removed. Other fruit spices include capsicums and chillies, fruits of various tropical perennials, large fruits being called capsicums and the smaller ones, chillies. There main use is as pickling spices. Cayenne pepper refers to the pungent powder produced by grinding mixtures of dried capsicums and chillies and is used in curries and spicy sauces. Paprika or Hungarian pepper, also comes from a dried ground capsicum and is less pungent while pimento, or allspice, is the dried unripe fruit of a species of myrtle.

The best-known seed spice, mustard, comes in two varieties, white and black, the white seed being three times the size of the black. Table mustard is made of a ground-up mixture of both varieties, plus turmeric for colour and wheat flour to absorb the essential oils. The powder is mixed with cold water, vinegar or oil, Whole mustard seeds are used for pickles and chutneys, Among the other seed spices are caraway, celery, coriander, mace and nutmeg. The latter two come from the same tree, mace being the dried husk around the kernel of the apricot-like fruit and nutmeg being the kernel itself.

From flowers we select cloves, the unopened buds of another tropical evergreen. Strongly aromatic, they add piquancy to fruit stews (notably apple) to sauces (such as bread sauce) and

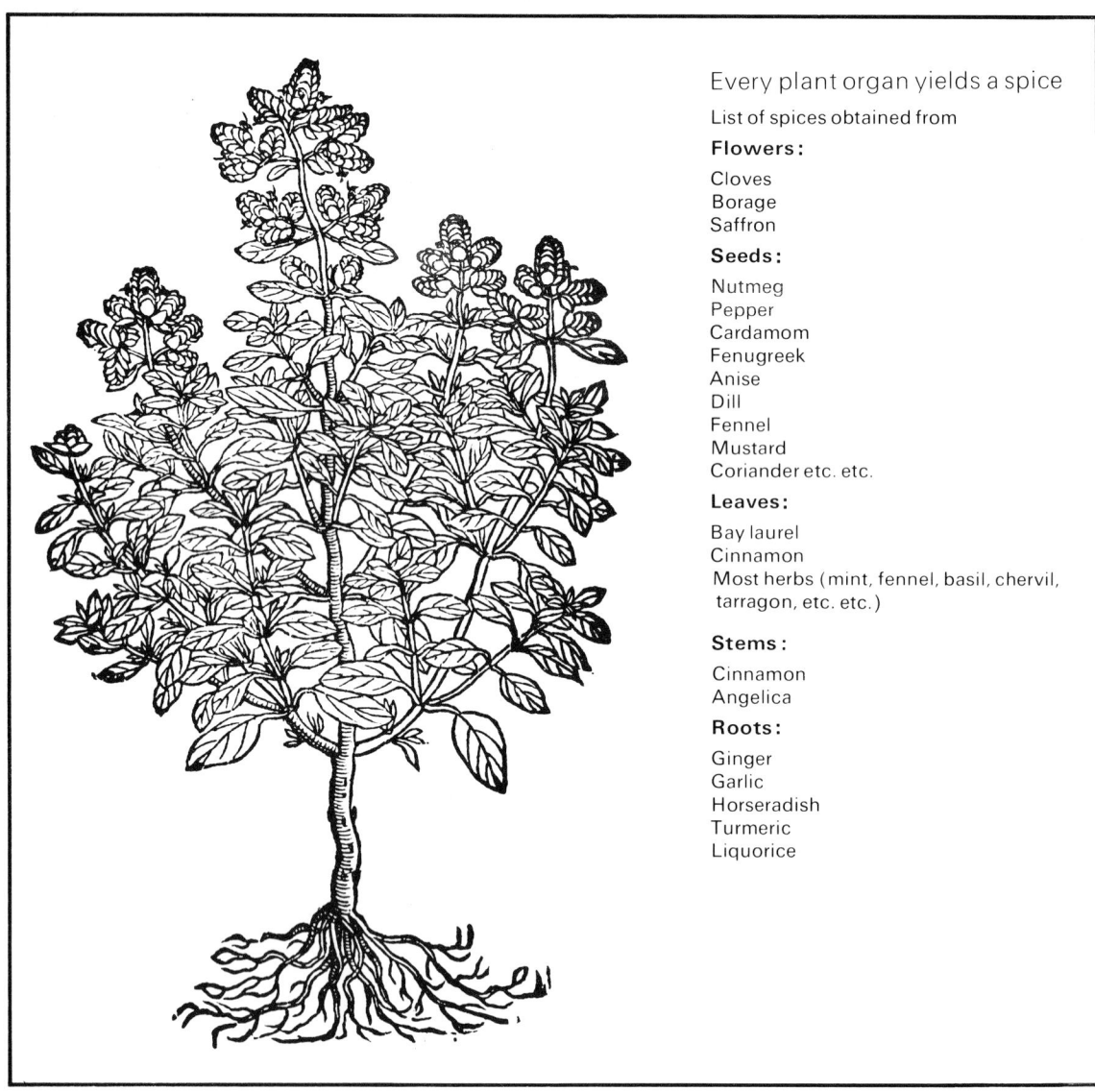

Every plant organ yields a spice

List of spices obtained from

Flowers:

Cloves
Borage
Saffron

Seeds:

Nutmeg
Pepper
Cardamom
Fenugreek
Anise
Dill
Fennel
Mustard
Coriander etc. etc.

Leaves:

Bay laurel
Cinnamon
Most herbs (mint, fennel, basil, chervil,
  tarragon, etc. etc.)

Stems:

Cinnamon
Angelica

Roots:

Ginger
Garlic
Horseradish
Turmeric
Liquorice

to pickles and chutneys. Saffron is the dried stigma and top of the saffron crocus, sometimes used in saffron cakes but more often seen by the public these days in the yellow tinted rice of proliferating Indian restaurants. Saffron Walden, in Essex, is apparently named after the saffron crocuses that were cultivated there in the 11th century, but the plant today is chiefly grown in Spain. The flower buds of a creeping shrub in the tropics, pickled in salt and vinegar, produce capers, superb with certain types of fish. Cinnamon, cassia and quinine are the chief bark spices. Cinnamon comes from an evergreen laurel grown in Sri Lanka and finds flavouring favour in cakes, puddings and pickles. Cassia is a similar, though inferior, product from another laurel and the bitter quinine, from the bark of the South American cinchona tree, is not only an effective anti-malarial drug but spices that bubbly tonic water drink by which *Sch . . . you know who*! made their name.

Finally, among the root spices are ginger, the rhizome (underground stem) of the herbaceous perennial *Zingiber officinale* or other members of the Zingiberaceae family. It adds sparkle to, or gingers up, a variety of foods. Turmeric comes from a somewhat similar plant and is used to give a rich yellowness to both mustard and curry powders. Curry powder itself is a mixture of spices, including coriander, chillies and cardamoms, ginger, nutmeg, peppers, pimentos and turmeric.

Those then are the main spices, the food additives that our grandfathers and our ancestors ate. In the early years of this century there was a decrease in their use, as bad-food disguises became less vital but there seems to have been a recent increase again as more home cooks turn to spices to flavour their efforts.

One doesn't hear of natural food faddists decrying such additives but it is no more natural to add mustard to beef than *monosodium glutamate* to soup.

The other ancient additives, many introduced into Britain by the Romans and by the various orders of monks, are the herbs. Often they were added to stews to mask the salty meat flavour or as stuffings, which served a similar purpose. The commonest are mint, parsley, sage and thyme, but others include aniseed, basil, bay, borage, chervil, chive, dill, fennel, garlic, horseradish, marjoram, rosemary and tarragon.

Mention was made earlier of Western man's aversion to insect eating, although many of the *insectae* are rich in protein. It seems a little strange, therefore, that we are quite happy to use material prepared from the dried carcasses of a cactus-eating insect. We use the unfortunate creature not as a nutrient, nor even as a flavour-enhancer, but merely as a scarlet dyestuff. It is called cochineal.

Perhaps one of the reasons we have accepted all these traditional additives is because they are 'natural products', not 'chemicals'. Their active ingredients, like the spices' essential oils or cochineal's scarlet carminic acid are, nonetheless, 'chemicals'. We can extract and isolate them and even recreate some of them synthetically.

Analysis shows, however, that these natural flavourings owe their subtlety not to any one substance but to a variety of different chemicals. It is easier, therefore, to use the natural product, rather than try to create the flavour artificially. But it is interesting to note that the main flavour of, for example, pineapple is *methyl-ß-methyl-thiol-propionate*. Strawberries gain much of their savour from *methylphenyl-glycidate*, onions from *ethyl thiocynate*, garlic from *diallyl disulphide* and mustard, from *allyl thiocarbimide*!

And some 'chemicals' have been used directly as additives for centuries. What else are the sodium nitrate or potassium nitrate (saltpetre) traditionally used to give hams and bacon their attractive red colour, but chemical additives?

Modern preservative and colouring additives

As well as the three traditional preservatives of salt, sugar and vinegar, chemical substances such as borax, *sodium benzoate*, *sodium salicylate* and formalin were shown to have germ-killing properties even in very small amounts. They were widely used but, because of the potential harmful effects, their use has been, since 1925, limited to certain products and controlled factory processes. Sodium benzoate and the chemically-related *benzoic acid*, for instance, are often added to margarine, to fruit juices and to pickles.

Other modern preservative additives include *sulphurous acid* and chemicals of the sulphite group which are added to fruit pulp which is ultimately to be made into jam. These potentially-hazardous substances are almost entirely vaporized during the jam boiling process. *Sodium diacetate*, *sodium and calcium propionates*, lactic acid and monocalcium phosphate are among the preservatives added to baked products; *sorbic acid* will inhibit the growth of moulds in cheese and *sulphur dioxide* is used to preserve dried fruits.

We should not forget also hops which, while added primarily as a flavouring, have strong antibacterial properties, fulfilling a valuable role in keeping our beer drinkable.

Also to be added to the list are those products which inhibit oxidation of foods, especially fats and oils, turning them rancid and foul-tasting. Among such anti-oxidants are acids, notably *ascorbic*, *citric*, *lactic*, *phosphoric* and *tartaric* which are added in concentrations of about one part per 15,000 of fat. They are, however, not greatly effective. Highly complex synthetic compounds are also used, among them *nordihydroguaiaretic acid* (NDGA) and *butylated hydroxyanisole* (BHA) and *butylated hydroxytoluene* (BHT). Incidentally both vitamin E and some of the spices, like chillies, turmeric and cinnamon also have anti-oxidant properties.

The importance of colour in stimulating appetite and the flow of the digestive juices has already been stated. In an effort to enhance the attractiveness of their wares, food producers and processors add a variety of colouring agents, all of which are now strictly controlled by law, specifically in Britain by the Colouring Matter in Food Regulations of 1957.

Most synthetic colours belong to the *diazo* group of organic compounds, derived from coal tar. Like Britain, most other countries have 'permitted lists' of colouring additives allowing only those that have been exhaustively tested and proved harmless to be used. Unfortunately we still seem to be far short of total international agreement on what artificial colours are to be allowed.

The trouble with the diazo compounds is that some of them may cause cancers in experimental animals, even in very small quantities, if given over long periods. The ones appearing in the various official lists have never been shown to be toxic in any way, but prudent food processors tend these days to rely more on naturally-occurring pigments, such as *carotene* (reddish-yellow dyes found in a number of vegetables as well as carrots), palm oil and *annatto*, an orange paste prepared from the fermented seed of the tropical *Bixa orellana* tree.

This might appear to be sensible but there is, of course, no guarantee that such 'natural' substances are any safer than synthetic ones. But it is disturbing that an additive permitted in one country may be considered hazardous in another and international agreement is to be hoped for.

As well as preserving and colouring, we add extras to our basic foods to improve their flavour; to 'improve' them, as in 'flour improvers'; to alter their texture, and to enhance their nutritional value.

Flavouring: the monosodium glutamate story

Here follows the curious case of a very widely used flavouring agent, *monosodium glutamate*, or MSG. Now the meat and yeast extracts we use for flavouring contain proteins which have been broken down into their constituent amino-acids. In 1908 a Japanese scientist discovered that one of the most effective flavourings within such melanges was *glutamic acid*. One of its salts,

monosodium glutamate provides an even more powerful meaty flavour. The Japanese, who manufacture it in great quantities, actually call it the 'essence of taste' and one of its curious properties is that of bringing out, or intensifying, the natural flavours of meats and chicken and other protein-rich foods such as fish and cheese. It is extensively used in soups, sauces, prepared meat dishes, fish products and even cheese spreads. So ubiquitous an additive is MSG that some 50 million pounds of it are used annually in the USA alone. And the active ingredient in soya sauce, that mainstay of Oriental cookery, is also MSG.

One must not forget that MSG or at least its acid, glutamic acid, is as 'natural' a product as you can get, for it is one of the products of protein breakdown within our bodies. The amounts we take in as a food additive are small compared with those we create after every meal.

Sixty years after MSG's isolation, however, an American doctor experienced nasty symptoms, including hot facial flushing of a temporary nature and headaches, after eating a Chinese meal. He wrote to a medical journal about it, wondered if other people had suffered similarly and dubbed his collection of symptoms the 'Chinese Restaurant Syndrome'.

It was fine copy for a rainy day and medical correspondents throughout the world – myself included – leaped on the story with glee but few people, I suspect, took it very seriously. It was quite possible that some people might be affected by extra-large doses of this amino-acid derivative, but surely the answer was to refrain from over-indulgence in Chinese food.

The doctor's letter, however, turned the spotlight on MSG and in one American research project very large doses – hundreds of times more than one would expect to ingest – were *injected* beneath the skin of mice; brain damage resulted.

As a result of this curious experiment, a number of American baby food manufacturers decided to withdraw MSG from their products. They still continued to use salt, however, although you will remember that rats fed the equivalent of one to two ounces of salt a day died at an age corresponding to 32 in man.

In the amounts present in most foods – about 0.1 to 0.3 per cent is the normal range – monosodium glutamate has never been shown to have any harmful or even unpleasant effect.

Other flavouring agents, even more powerful than MSG in bringing out the meatiness or tastiness of protein foods are the ribonucleolides, derivatives of another very natural product, ribonucleic acid or RNA. Prepared from yeast extracts, the ribonucleolides are either used separately or in combination with monosodium glutamate.

Other uses of additives

Over the years many different substances have been added to bread and controversy still reigns today over what should be added, or what not taken away. The arguments are analysed in Chapter Six. One group of bread additives – the so-called 'flour improvers' – however, fit more properly into this section. These improvers are added to flour to produce a bigger, stronger and more open-textured loaf. We are not sure how they work but it seems they encourage the linking up of certain protein chains within the dough.

In 1919 a very powerful improver, *nitrogen trichloride* gas, was introduced. Known commercially as 'Agene' it was the most widely utilised flour improver until, in 1946, it was shown that dogs fed on large amounts of Agene-treated flour developed fits apparently due to a substance formed by the action of the gas on one of the amino-acids in the flour. Extensive tests on humans failed to demonstrate that the product produced any harmful effects on man but nonetheless Agene was withdrawn and its use is forbidden. Chlorine dioxide – 'Dyox' – is now commonly used instead. As well as being an improver it also acts as a bleach, producing a whiter loaf.

For the full enjoyment of food texture is as important as taste, smell and colour. Watery sauces and soups, for example, are distinctly unappetising, so starch is widely used as a thickening agent. Heating starch in water causes the granules to swell and gelatinise, forming a thick paste. Canned soups, dried soup powders and 'instant' sauces all contain starch.

For other foods, we insist on a 'creamy' texture and to achieve this we often need another type of additive, the *emulsifier*. Anyone who has tried to make mayonnaise will know that oil and water – or in this case, oil and vinegar – will not mix. You may shake them together but they soon separate into their own sections. Egg yolk acts as an emulsifier to bind them both together in a smooth mixture, although producing the emulsion by hand may be a tricky business.

Many of our foods, such as ice-cream and margarine are water and oil or water and fat mixtures and they too need emulsifying agents to achieve an acceptable degree of smoothness. There are many emulsifiers and they are widely used but the most popular of all is *glycerol monostearate* or GMS which has almost completely replaced older 'natural' emulsifiers like the *lecithin* in egg yolk. Those who decry such a trend can take comfort from the fact that in the body it is broken down into glycerol and stearic acid, two of the breakdown products of 'natural' fats.

Finally, there are the nutritive additives, such as the B-group vitamins added to bread (see Chapter Six), the vitamins A and D added to margarine, the variety of vitamins and minerals in our cornflakes and the extra vitamin C mixed in with many fruit drinks and juices. Incidentally, it is worth mentioning that wholly-synthetic vitamin C is usually added and there are those who believe this is inferior to the natural product. Chemically and nutritionally, however, there is absolutely no difference.

This is not the place to become embroiled in the continuing debate about another additive, *fluoride*, which helps protect children's teeth and occurs naturally in many water supplies in concentrations far in excess of those artificially-induced by local authorities concerned with preventive medicine. But it is interesting that a related salt – iodide – is added to salt to protect those in low-iodine areas from goitre.

As far as nutritive additives are concerned, it *is* possible to have too much of a good thing, as we found out in Britain when we added vitamin D (calciferol) to our National Dried Milk. We erred on the side of generosity to make sure every baby received enough of the anti-rickets vitamin and to compensate for any losses in processing and storage. While rickets certainly all but disappeared, the high dose of vitamin D precipitated cases of another disease, *hypercalcaemia* – that is excess calcium in the blood, which disturbs the function of nerve and muscle cells. Calciferol levels were quickly reduced.

Mention ought also to be made of unwanted or unintentional additives, not just the odd cigarette butt, button or dead mouse in processed food (still occasional occurrences despite the efforts of Public Health Inspectors) but the more insidious infiltration of pesticides, notably DDT. Now, no person that we know of has ever died of DDT ingestion, even though one pesticide factory worker once ate pounds of the stuff. But it was a sobering thought that in the late 1960s and early 1970s the average man in the USA had a higher concentration of DDT in his bloodstream than was legally permitted in the meat he could buy.

In Britain levels were about a quarter as high, at about one hundredth of an ounce per person. Nonetheless there was strong evidence that DDT and a number of other widely-used pesticides were killing off animal life, from micro-organisms and plankton to birds of prey. Most countries either ban their use completely or impose the strictest of controls.

The search for safety

As we have seen, in the search for safety those testing the additives for our food insist on an extremely large margin for error. It is a general rule that the poor old experimental animal must eat 100 times as much of a new additive as will ever be used in practice, for its entire lifetime – and two generations of its offspring do the same – without demonstrable harm. As far as cancer is concerned the American Panel on Food Additives of the President's Science Advisory Committee recommended a few years ago that a substance could be cleared of potential carcinogenicity at certain dose levels if no malignant tumours developed in 1000 test animals. Statistical analysis of this recommendation, however, showed that even a substance capable of causing 100,000 cases of cancer among the US population would have a one in three chance of being cleared by such a test. It should be remembered too that the response to different substances varies between animal species, and between animals and man. (It is interesting to note here that had the stringent testing procedures now insisted on for drugs been applied to penicillin, that great life saver would never have been passed for human use. It is toxic to guinea pigs but has no such effect in humans.)

There can never be such a thing as absolute safety; we can only make an assessment of possible risks and try to ensure they are reduced to an absolute minimum.

The issues over additives have been clouded by emotionalism and ill-formed concepts of natural and synthetic foods. Of course it is right to insist on the highest standards of testing before adding anything new to our foods. But the results of such tests must be examined with extreme care to ensure we do not place the wrong, alarmist interpretations on them.

Whatever our feelings, too, we may be sure that additives are here to stay. Not counting sugar or salt, in 1974 each of us swallowed some three pounds of them and the amount seems to be rising inexorably. All in all there are at least 2500 various types. Such a statistic is often quoted with horror but when one examines what additives are used for and what sort of substances they are, they really become far less frightening than those who call for 'natural' foods would have us believe.

4 How natural is natural? Food Processing

'By the end of August the frozen food industry will have packed and stored another 400 million packets of peas and beans – enough to keep the shopkeepers' cabinets stocked for the next 12 months. [Food freezing] has grown into an £800 million industry with a chain of low temperature storage depots linking 130,000 shops to the hundreds of producers who supply them. This 'cold chain' extends today into three million homes – three million kitchens with home freezers.'

Special Report on Frozen Foods, 'The Times', August 4th, 1975.

'It has been predicted that by 1980 no less than 80 per cent of all the housewife's food purchases will be in convenience form. According to a 1970 survey carried out by Unigate foods, spending on convenience foods will double between 1970 and 1980.'

Allan Cameron on 'Instant Food' in 'Food – Facts and Fallacies'.

'Part of the secret of success in life is to eat what you like and let the food fight it out inside.'

Mark Twain.

In the factory at Great Yarmouth where food freezing began in Britain 30 years ago they now freeze in 24 hours as many peas and beans as they did in the whole of the 1945 season: food processing really has become big business.

It is not just freezing, of course. An extraordinarily wide variety of techniques have evolved for preserving food, for enhancing its flavour and altering its texture and, perhaps above all, for presenting it in a form that is simple to prepare and straightforward to cook and serve.

This chapter is about food processing and why the term 'processed food' seems to have become a pejorative one. For, just as traditional food additives have been unquestioned and uncriticised, yet modern ones condemned, so too are traditional processing methods acceptable and 'natural' yet latter-day techniques often condemned as unwholesome and artificial.

It is a curious phenomenon that while with almost any other product the word 'new' will enhance its reputation ('new', improved washing powders, 'new' hi-fi electronics, for example), perhaps the worst way of promoting food products is to describe them as new foods. As far as food is concerned familiarity seems to breed content – and this can cause not a few headaches for the advertising man trying to promote a novel food product.

In an entertaining *Sunday Times* analysis of this ingrained distrust of novelty, Michael Bateman wrote that the advertiser is concerned with generating excitement about his products but 'he has to confess that you cannot do this in food by proclaiming its novelty'. He quotes Jeremy Bullmore, creative director of Britain's biggest advertising agents, J. Walter Thompson: 'People are apprehensive about new things which are by definition untried and unknown. It is one thing to say New Oxo, which means the same old Oxo only slightly different. But if you are talking about the Batemanburger, made out of soya beans, that's different.'

So a variety of highly-sophisticated techniques have been evolved to persuade us to buy new foods, or foods prepared in new ways. Margarine is a classic example: would you have eaten hydrogenated palm, coconut and herring oil if you had not been persuaded that it looked like, felt like and tasted like butter? Much food advertising, as we shall see, has little to do, with hunger or nutritional requirements, and in its highly-expensive, invasive promotion of its products the food industry has been subjected to a great deal of, often justified, criticism.

Another reason why food processing seems to have gained a bad reputation is because of its scale. Surely, it is argued, mass factory production line techniques must be inferior to the efforts of a skilled chef. Certainly many of the ways of treating food on an industrial scale are far removed from the 'cottage industry' style of the restaurant or home kitchen.

But what is the matter with food processing? Are true tastes and textures being destroyed? Are valuable or even vital nutrients being lost?

As we saw in Chapters One and Three, there is no such thing as a natural food for Man – and nor is there such a thing as the natural state in which our food should be eaten. In fact, from the earliest times we have been processing our food, for the most radical food process of all is cooking.

The cooking process

We do not know when man first learned how to start a fire but it is certainly one of the earliest and most universal of all human discoveries. Man, it has been said, is scarcely man until he is in possession of fire – and no fireless tribe of men has even been found anywhere in the world. It is likely that the first use of this precious gift was in keeping warm or frightening off wild animals but it cannot have been long before the advantages of applying heat to food were realised.

Did a hunk of mastodon steak fall accidentally into the fire? Or was a lump of meat skewered by some early Escoffier and experimentally toasted over the flames? No matter what the answers to such conjectures, it is cooking his food that sets civilised man apart from the other animals, all of which eat their food raw.

Processing food by heat confers a number of advantages: it 'tenderises' making eating and digestion easier; it develops new flavours which stimulate the appetite; it enhances the appeal to senses other than taste by improving appearance and releasing appetising aromas; and, it destroys germs and the micro-organisms of decay.

While ancient man may have existed well enough on raw meat, eggs, fish and wild fruit and berries, once he had learned the secret of cooking there was no going back. And as well as merely heating his food in air man learned the further

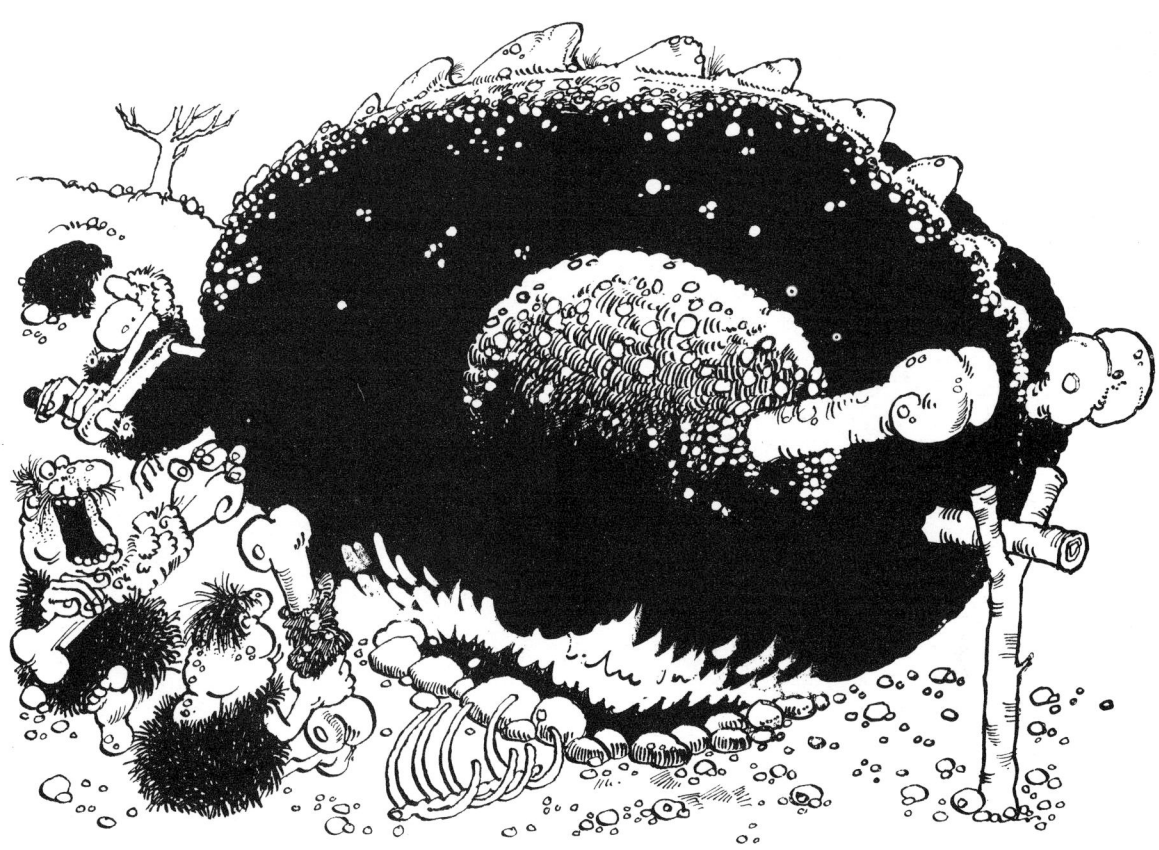

"It is cooking his food that sets man apart . . ."

advantages of moist heat in stewing, boiling and steaming and of the high temperatures obtained by frying in hot fat.

We enjoy cooked food because of its stimulation of the senses in enhanced flavour, texture, appearance and smell, but cooking confers other benefits as well. For a start, it is essential for the digestion of starch. As we have seen in Chapter Two, starch in such foods as cereals and flour, potatoes and rice is locked in granules which are almost impenetrable by the digestive juices. In cooking with moist heat both the cellulose and starch components are softened by the absorption of water. Further cooking produces no other changes in the cellulose but causes a swelling and *gelatinisation* of the starch molecules. The starch changes from hard lumps to a softer jelly. This the digestive juices can easily break down into glucose for absorption into the bloodstream. Such gelatinisation takes place when potatoes or rice are boiled and when bread is baked.

Changes occur also in the *pectin*, a complex polysaccharide which reinforces the cellulose cell walls in fruit and vegetables. This is converted by hot water into a softer, more soluble form. The softer texture of boiled potatoes compared with roast potatoes, for example, is due to the fact that more of this soluble pectin is dissolved in water, enabling more gelatinisation of starch.

Advantages of cooking

Proteins are coagulated by cooking, a process most easily visible in the conversion of the runny transparent part of an egg to a firmer white on boiling. This process occurs in other proteins too. The lean part of meat is muscle, composed of bundles of parallel fibres sheathed in connective tissue and held together by a type of protein called *collagen*.

In cooking this collagen first coagulates and then is converted by the water present in the meat

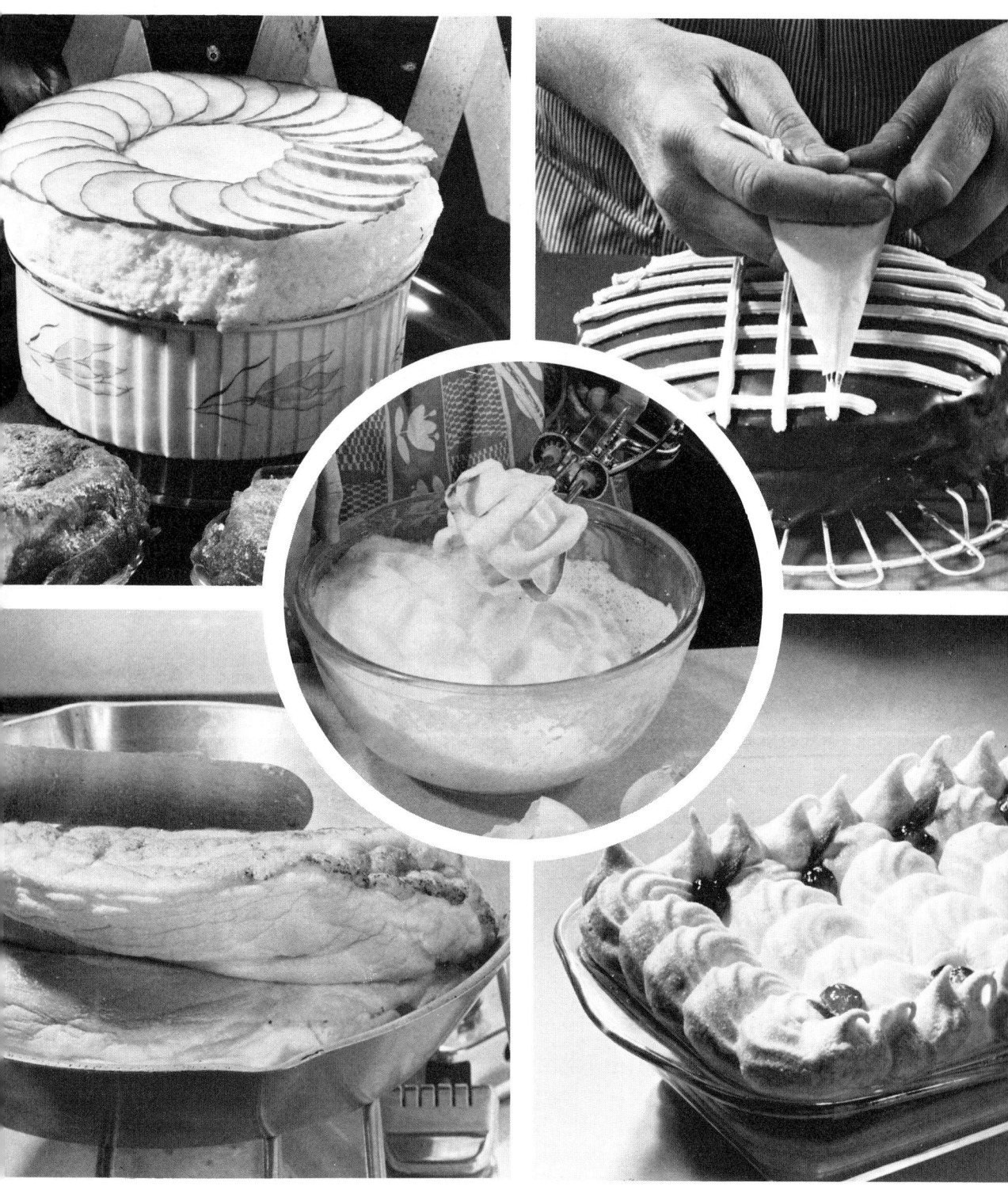

Beaten egg as a basic construction material.

into soft, gelatin, which is further melted by the heat. Some of the resulting fluid mixture seeps out of the meat and in a roast much of it dries on the outside, while in a stew it mixes with the added water and other ingredients.

This breakdown of collagen and its dropping away as gelatin causes shrinkage of the meat and this process is further accelerated by a breakdown and coagulation of the proteins that form the muscle fibres themselves, which begins to occur at a temperature of about 60°C (140°F). The net effect of all these chemical changes is that the muscle fibres become shorter and more brittle, and they separate much more easily. They are consequently easier to chew, and simpler to digest.

Incidentally, cooked meat changes in colour from red to brown because of a pigment in the muscle fibres called *myoglobin* (closely related to the *haemoglobin* pigment in the blood). When heated, the iron atoms in the pigment become permanently oxidised changing to a brown colour. It is merely a coincidence that this change occurs at about the same temperature as the muscle fibre proteins are broken down (around 60°C) so that browning indicates that the meat is cooked.

One other advantage of cooking is more of a side-effect than a direct benefit: it can sometimes increase the amounts of minerals in our diet. Calcium may be absorbed from hard water into the food, and iron from the utensils!

In many instances, then, cooking enhances the quality of our food, making it more appetising and easier to eat and digest. Some foods, of course, are better raw and whatever processing technique is applied, it fails to retain the original qualities. Strawberries are an obvious example: in the canning process they have to be cooked (see page 67) and this ruins the texture which is so essential a part of our enjoyment of the fruit. Freezing, too, can destroy the strawberry's delicate cellular framework so that it does not feel as it ought in the mouth.

Another disadvantage of the cooking process, whether at home or in the factory is that it can destroy a high proportion of certain nutrients, particularly Vitamin C.

Preventing the loss of Vitamin C

Vitamin C is destroyed by heat and is also extremely soluble in water. A further problem is

that enzymes within the plant cells also gradually destroy the vitamin. Stored potatoes, for example, are a reasonable source in the autumn but by the spring there will be little vitamin C left. And vitamin C is easily destroyed by air, too, so the fresher the vegetable the better. Mashing potatoes, which greatly increases the surface area in contact with the air, can also lead to considerable losses.

All in all it is reckoned that the average loss in boiling peeled potatoes is around 50 per cent. Frying, baking or boiling in their skin reduces the vitamin C loss considerably. Cabbage, cauliflower, brussels sprouts, peas and runner beans are all susceptible to losses of 50 per cent and more, and with kale as much as 85 per cent of the vitamin C originally present may be lost in the cooking process.

There are a number of ways to reduce these losses. As little water as possible should be used and the vegetables boiled vigorously (this destroys the enzyme) but for the shortest possible time. It also helps to cut the vegetables into larger pieces rather than grate them and to serve them as soon as possible after cooking.

Other cooking losses

Some of the B-group of vitamins are susceptible to heat, too. Thiamine, for example, is almost all lost in baking biscuits. Only about 8 per cent is lost in baking bread with yeast, but when soda is added the loss can approach 100 per cent. In wholemeal bread, although the thiamine content is initially higher there still may be losses of up to 35 per cent, even if yeast is used. And more thiamine may be destroyed by the very high temperatures needed to make toast.

How to keep your Vitamin C when cooking

Vitamin C is destroyed by exposure to air and heat, and it dissolves in water, so in cooking you need to:

1 Use the *least possible* water.
2 Bring it to the boil.
3 Put in your greens (having *just* chopped them, where necessary).
4 Cook *fast* until just tender enough.
5 Serve *as soon as possible* – and *use* the water that's left.
6 **Never** use bicarbonate – it makes a nice green colour but it's death to vitamin C.

There may be some loss of minerals during cooking but these are unlikely to be significant.

The advantages of cooking, particularly in gelatinising the starch ready for digestion, outweigh the disadvantages of vitamin loss. And careful cooking can ensure that even these losses can be kept to a minimum.

So far we have been examining 'food processing' in a domestic or semi-domestic sense. Mass food processing may occasionally be an extension and adaptation of home procedures on much larger scale, but often it uses completely different techniques which would be impossible or impractical at home.

One ancient process that has largely passed from home to factory is bread-making, but the arguments over this processing of flour to make it palatable are discussed elsewhere (see Chapter Six).

As we have seen when looking at additives, one of the greatest problems our forebears had with their food was preserving it from decay through the long winters. In their attempts to keep their food edible they used salt, sugar and vinegar as preservatives and they were liberal with their use of spices to disguise the taste of salt and the smell of decay.

It was not until Pasteur's discoveries in the second half of the last century that the culprits responsible for putrefaction were identified. They are micro-organisms, or germs, notably bacteria and moulds which live off the food and contaminate it with various breakdown products and acids, so that it eventually putrefies. Like most living things, however, they are susceptible to extremes of heat and cold, and to a lack of water. Food preservation techniques exploit these susceptibilities.

Bottling and canning

The first modern processes for preservation were developed empirically some half a century before the true cause of food spoilage was known. In 1795 the embryonic revolutionary republic of France was beset by enemies on all sides and the government was desperate to seek better ways of preserving food for its troops. (As Napoleon said, an army marches on its stomach.)

A prize of 12,000 francs was offered and it was won, after many years patient experimentation by a Parisian confectioner Nicolas Appert. He published, in 1810, *The Book for All Households*

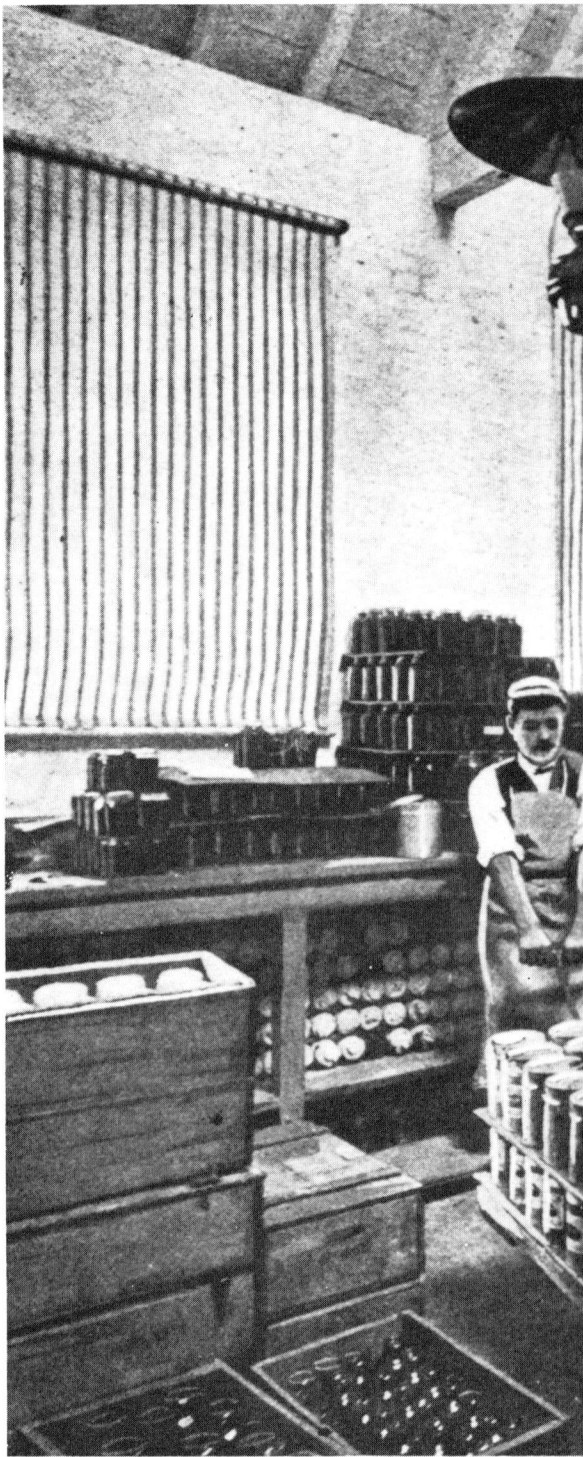

A jam factory in the 19th Century.

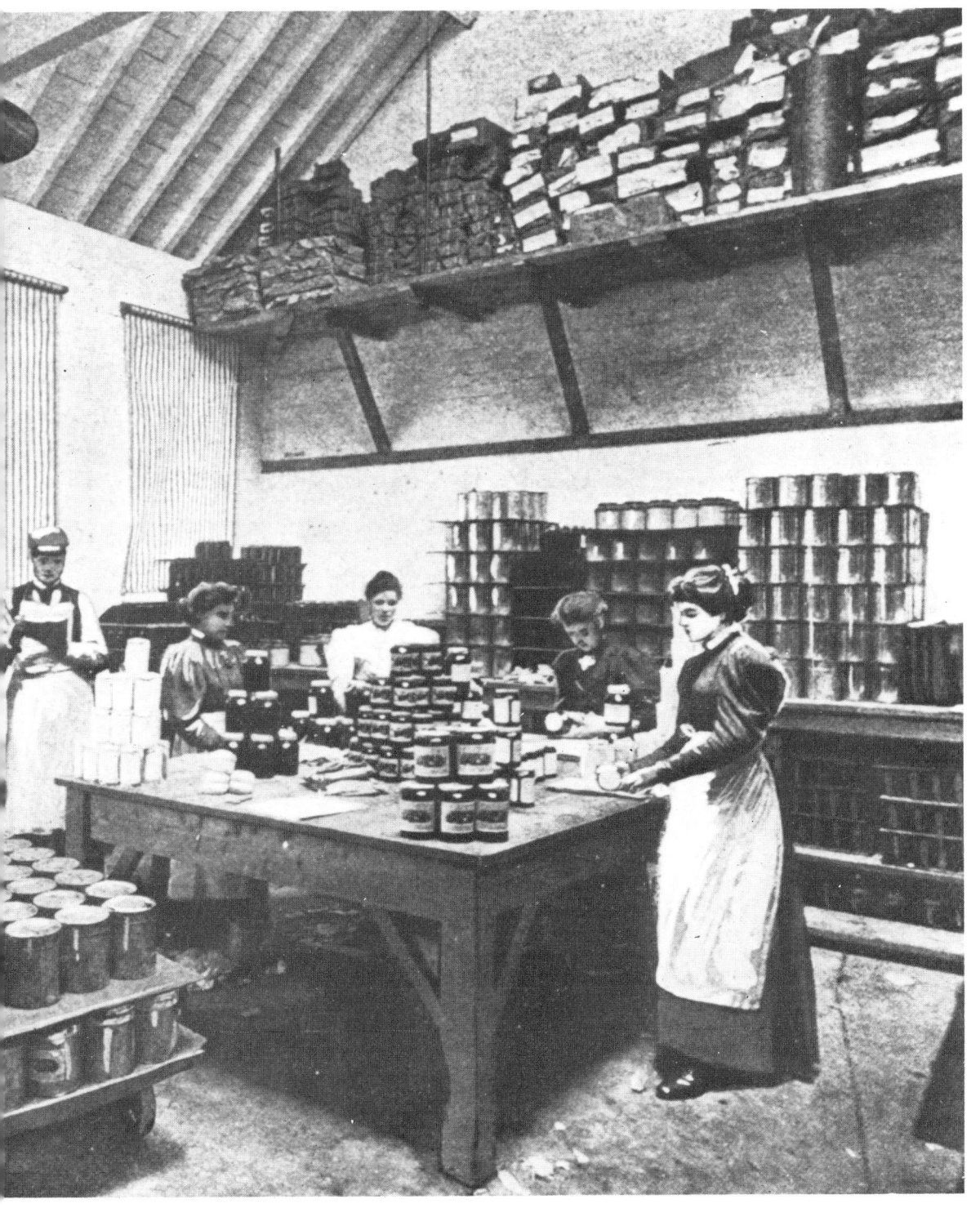

E

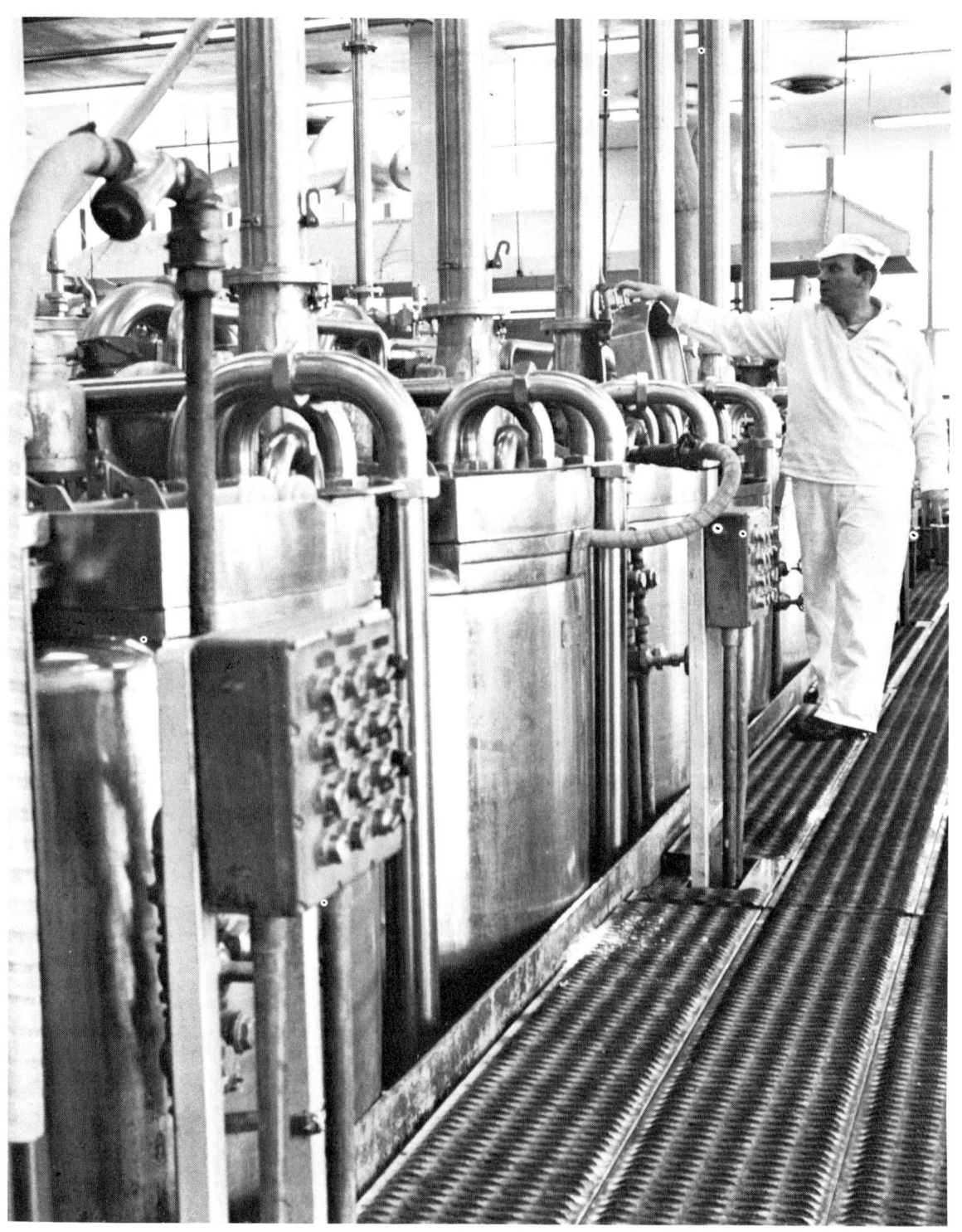

A modern cannery.

on The Art of Preserving Animal Substances for Many Years giving details of the bottling process he had discovered.

Placing food in glass bottles, Appert covered it with water and then cooked for several hours. The bottles were then hermetically sealed with waxed corks which were wired onto the bottles.

Although there have been many improvements in techniques over the years, the principles underlying bottling – and canning too, for it is basically the same method – have remained unaltered. The heat kills off almost all the micro-organisms, and the spores by which they spread. The sealing prevents any fresh germs entering and contaminating the food.

Bottling or canning does not reach absolute sterility, because some spores are extraordinarily resistant: the modern canner or bottler first ensures that all pathogenic organisms, that is those that cause disease, are destroyed. The most potent of these are *Salmonella*, *Staphylococcus* and *Clostridium* organisms, all of which can produce severe food poisoning and even kill. Then the canner must try to kill off as many 'spoilage' organisms as he can, without destroying the texture and flavour of the food by over-cooking. He is able to achieve a large measure of success and the few organisms which survive are mostly those called *thermophiles* – they love heat – which will not multiply under normal storage conditions.

Cans soon replaced bottles, the earliest ones being handmade and having a hole in the lid which was sealed with a solder plug when the can was still hot.

In a modern canning factory the food is first cleaned and prepared – fruit and vegetables washed, meat removed from bone and chopped up etc. – and then blanched by being immersed in boiling water or surrounded by steam. This is especially important for vegetables such as peas, for it drives out air bubbles trapped within their structures. It can also improve flavour and texture and destroys enzymes which might affect the food's long-term stability.

Meat or fish may be cooked or compressed before canning and sometimes hot products are poured directly into the cans from the cookers. It is usually cold, however, and the filling is done automatically and at high speed. Filled cans pass to an 'exhaust box' where exposure to hot water or steam immediately before sealing the lid creates an air-free vacuum at the top of the can. Sealing, too,

is very rapid, machines being capable of hermetically covering 250 or more cans a minute.

The cooking time depends on a number of factors including the size of the can and the acidity of the contents. Fruits, for example, are generally acidic and since bacteria cannot grow in an acid environment it is necessary only to kill off yeasts and moulds. This can be done by heating the cans to boiling point (100°C) for some 10 to 15 minutes. For non-acid foods higher temperatures are needed – at least 116°C – and this is usually achieved by putting the cans in an autoclave (a large pressure cooker) and heating with pressurised steam.

There are disadvantages with such techniques. Even in an autoclave, the time taken for cooking can mean a loss of vitamins from the food and a deterioration in flavour or texture. This can be overcome by a method known as aseptic canning applied to liquid and semi-liquid foods. Here the food itself is passed through a heat exchanger (usually a system of pipes) where it is rapidly heated for a period which may vary from just a few seconds to several minutes, and then immediately cooled down again. The sterilised food is put into cans (themselves pre-sterilised) and hermetically sealed.

Sheet steel is used for the cans and there is an extremely thin lining of tin to prevent any chemical reaction between food and can. For acid-containing foods, further protection is given by lacquering or enamelling the can's inside.

Preserving and purifying milk: Pasteurisation

Cow's milk is an excellent and widely-used foodstuff. It is the nearest thing we have to a perfect food, being an exceptionally good source of protein, one of the best sources of calcium and containing a wide selection of essential vitamins, notably A, D and a number from the B group. In developed countries the milk industry is now highly organised, bringing to our doorsteps a daily 'pinta' with the minimum of delay.

Unfortunately, as well as being so nutritious a food for humans, milk is also an ideal breeding ground for bacteria and the chain of events in bringing it from cow to doorstep allow many opportunities to introduce microbes which can lead to spoilage. The problem lies not so much with the cow itself but with dirty cowsheds, unhygienic milkers, and milking equipment, and careless transport and processing.

Considerable effort is expended these days to ensure that all milking, bottling and transport procedures are hygienically carried out. It is still, however, essential to make sure that any microbes in the milk are either totally destroyed or so severely curtailed as to be harmless.

The microbes can be completely destroyed by sterilisation, heating the milk to at least 100°C and holding it at that temperature for some time. In commercial practice a common procedure is to load milk-filled bottles (with a screw or spring clip top) into a pressure vessel and raise the temperature to some 110°C for about 15 minutes. The trouble with sterilisation is that it alters both the taste and texture of the milk: some of the protein is cooked, the fine emulsion of fat is broken up and some 50 per cent of the vitamin C and much of the vitamin B_1 is destroyed.

These changes are to a large extent, however, dependent on time and a newer sterilisation process overcomes many of the difficulties. It is called the UHT or *ultra high temperature* process and produces a 'long life milk' capable of being kept for six months at ordinary room temperatures without going off. There is also far less destruction of vitamins and effect on taste.

In the UHT system fresh milk is heated to 132°C for just one second, which effectively sterilises it. The milk may be passed through a heat exchanger or have superheated steam injected directly into it.

Although we talk of 'sterilisation' even these processes do not achieve absolute destruction of every bacterium or spore. The milk *will* keep safely for many months, but not indefinitely.

The Pasteurisation process was originally developed by Louis Pasteur in the middle of the 19th century for destroying organisms in wine. Now widely used to treat milk, pasteurisation kills off virulent microbes, leaves taste unaltered and extends the life of the milk by a few days.

There are two pasteurisation techniques: the 'holder process' and 'flash pasteurisation'. In the former, the milk is heated to 63°C to 65°C and held there for 30 minutes. In flash pasteurisation the milk is heated to 72°C but this temperature is held for only 15 seconds before cooling begins. Of course, it is not just spoilage brought on by microbes that is of concern when milk is sold. There may be virulent microbes present, too, such

as tuberculosis bacilli and the organisms responsible for brucellosis and scarlet fever. These, and any organisms accidentally introduced in handling and processing are all destroyed by pasteurisation as well as most of the 'milk souring' organisms.

Apart from these beneficial effects, the process brings about only one other significant change: it does reduce vitamin C content. But it should be emphasised that milk is low in vitamin C anyway and even unpasteurised milk will not provide adequate dietary amounts of the vitamin.

Despite its obvious benefits, there was widespread and bitter controversy in the 1930s about the pasteurisation of milk. It was an argument which, in many ways, crystallised the 'natural' versus 'processed' foods debate, and the fight against pasteurisation continued for a number of years.

The main plank of the protesters' argument seemed to be that cows' milk had been specially created as a natural food for man and that to interfere with it was not only harmful but somehow sinful as well. A variety of scientific, or pseudo-scientific arguments were brought into play. In 1942, Professor G. S. Wilson summed up the objectors' claims: 'Pasteurisation diminishes the nutritive value of milk . . . it affects the taste and palatability, it affects the cream line, it reduces the amounts of calcium and phosphates, it

Making Yoghourt simply

Yoghourt is simply milk that has been soured by a particular bacterium. This causes it to set, and gives it a pleasant acid flavour. To make it:

1 You need to kill the other bacteria in your milk, so *just* bring it to the boil.

2 The yoghourt bacteria grow best about blood heat, so cool the hot milk, *then*

3 Add about 1 dessertspoon per pint of commercial yoghourt (or some from a friend).

4 Mix thoroughly.

5 Put in a closed container and *keep* it *warm*. Either wrap it up or put it in an airing cupboard or other warm place.

6 In a few hours, more or less as it is warmer or cooler, it will set to a nice smooth consistency. If it is left too long, the liquid separates and it looks unpleasant.

7 Once made, keep it in the refrigerator, so that the process will not go too far.

Of course, you also can do it conveniently with a commercial electrically warmed yoghourt-maker, or even with a large vacuum jar.

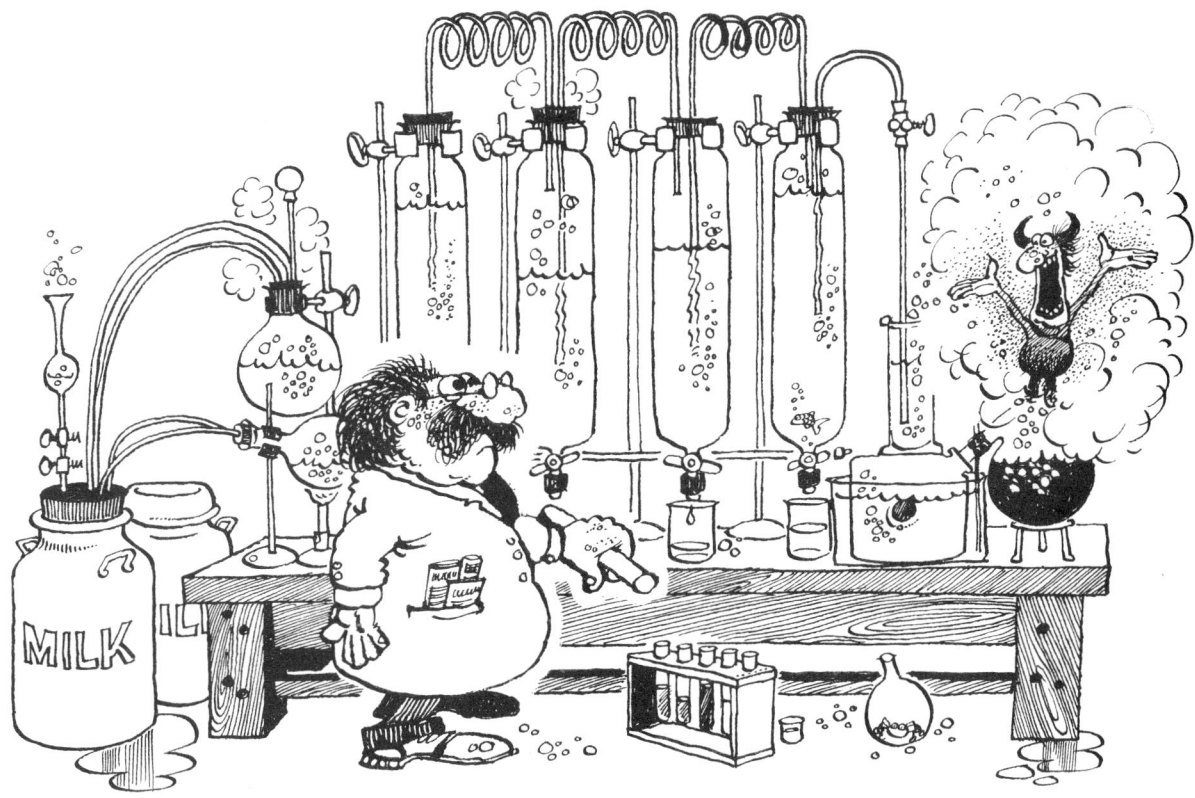

"To interfere with milk was somehow sinful . . ."

causes protein to coagulate at five degrees higher temperature, it destroys vitamin C, B vitamins, vitamin D and vitamin E.'

Wilson dismissed the first three claims as irrelevant, and in fact the effect on milk's chemical composition or flavour are minimal. As far as the cream line is concerned, the immediate cooling of milk after the pasteurisation process ensures that the amount of cream hardly changes at all. Calcium and phosphates are *not* affected, Wilson pointed out, and the protein coagulation point is utterly irrelevant.

The vitamin loss arguments, except for vitamin C, are false too, and as we have seen adults do not depend on milk for their vitamin C supplies and children are better off with safe milk, and orange juice for their vitamin C.

There is another argument against pasteurisation, that it will reduce resistance to disease. True, immunity to infections is built up by contracting the infection and producing antibodies against it in the blood, so that a fresh attack by the same type of invader will be immediately repulsed. The trouble is tuberculosis was potentially fatal and frequently crippling and brucellosis still remains a chronic disease which is extraordinarily difficult to treat successfully. So unpasteurised milk can be a killer – and there is no epidemiological evidence to suggest that it does in fact help disease resistance.

Another canard was that pasteurised milk could make children more prone to dental decay. This surprising assertion was based on a research report which commented on the excellent teeth of some boys in an institution where the milk supply was not pasteurised. No comparison was made with any group of similar boys drinking pasteurised milk, and again all the epidemiological evidence failed to uphold such claims.

Lastly, it was suggested that pasteurisation would diminish the incentive of dairies and bottling plants to work under hygienic conditions.

69

The evidence of the last 40 years, where the trend has been towards the highest possible standards of sterility and hygiene, has belied this piece of sophistry.

The pasteurisation controversy has much in common with current arguments about fluoridation, so it is easy for us to understand how it was able to continue for a decade or more before rationality overcame emotion. It required a considerable amount of research effort with large surveys involving thousands of children, whose health and growth was meticulously measured. None of the surveys showed any differences in the nutritive value of the two types of milk.

As Magnus Pyke says in his book *Food and Society*: 'The argument about the value of milk pasteurisation is now ended. In Great Britain the logic of the process was finally accepted by the nation in World War II – as the logic of votes for women had been in World War I.

'The conclusion came when the British citizens found that American soldiers based in England were not permitted to drink the local milk supply because no assurance could be given that it was properly free from infection.'

Of course, many of the arguments derived not from scientific certainty that pasteurisation was harmful, but from an emotional conviction that 'natural is best'. Such feelings still apply to attitudes to all kinds of food processing.

As far as pasteurisation is concerned, perhaps the last word should be left to Professor K. S. Kon, writing in *Nutritional Review* in 1967: 'What is a natural food for an omnivorous animal such as man I have never been able to understand, nor could I perceive why it should be more unnatural to heat a cow's milk than to cook her flesh.'

Preservation by drying

Drying food is one of the oldest methods of preservation. Micro-organisms need moisture to thrive. Additionally, the drying concentrates soluble substances in the food and this too inhibits the growth of bacteria, yeasts and moulds. (A classic example is the high sugar content of dried dates.) Natural enzymes, which act as catalysts in the breakdown processes which contribute to decay, are also unable to act in the absence of water.

Unlike preservation by heat, however, drying does not *destroy* either the microbes or the enzymes. When water is re-introduced they can soon become active again.

The oldest technique in drying, of course, was simply to leave the food in question out in the sun. Methods have now become industrialised and there are several different ways in which the moisture can be extracted. In the commonest system food on perforated trays passes through a chamber where hot air is blown over it with fans. An even simpler technique uses a kiln where warm air passes up through the food to be dried. Liquids are dried by being poured slowly over a heated, revolving horizontal cylinder. They dry almost instantly and are scraped off the roller. There is also a process called 'spray drying' whereby liquids are pumped downwards in a fine spray through which hot air is blown upwards. The droplets dry immediately and fall to the floor as powder.

Both roller-drying and spray-drying are particularly used for milk. The latter has advantages in that it is totally resoluble in water. With roller-dried milk there is invariably a small amount of insoluble residue left when the milk is reconstituted. It is, however, less bulky, so is easier to pack, store and transport.

Dehydration is used for preserving vegetables – dried peas are an obvious example – and potatoes, but cooked meat and fish can also be dehydrated and reconstituted when needed into nutritious foods.

When vegetables are to be dehydrated they must first be 'blanched', that is scalded for a short time in boiling water or steam. This prevents enzyme activity which would not only lead to large losses of vitamin C but also affect flavour and colour when vegetables are dried. Commercially, a small amount of *sodium sulphite* is also added to the scalding water, helping to preserve still further colour and vitamin C levels.

Dehydration of potatoes is used to make those packets of 'instant mash'. The cooked potato is machine mashed and then only partially dried, until its moisture content falls to about 50 per cent of the original. It is then allowed to cool for a couple of hours, a 'conditioning' process which produces a finer powder after the final drying. The partially-dried mash is sieved and then dried in trays exposed to hot air until moisture levels drop to about 5 per cent.

Reconstituted mashed potato has approximately

the same nutritive value as the natural product. Although vitamin C is lost during dehydration, synthetic vitamin C is often added after drying.

The latest development in instant mashed potatoes is dehydrated lumps or granules, rather than powder. These are said to improve the texture of the reconstituted mash. They are made by a technique called agglomeration in which the potato powder is reformed into lumps. (The exact procedures are closely guarded secrets of the manufacturers.)

Older factory dehydration techniques were fairly slow and this led to a loss of nutrients and quality. The latest techniques use lower temperatures and exclude oxygen (vacuum drying) which improves quality.

But all dehydration techniques are really only sophisticated variations on the age-old practices of leaving foods to dry in the sun. The most modern drying method, however, utilises a rather different principle. It is called freeze-drying.

Freeze-drying: drying from the frozen state

Basically, freeze-drying consists of quickly freezing the moisture in the product and then directly drying out or draining out the ice without it going through its liquid stage. The ice is removed by placing the frozen food in a high vacuum chamber. This causes direct evaporation to a vapour without any intermediate liquid stage. Incidentally a similar process occurs when washing is hung out to dry on very cold days. The washing can freeze but then be dried out by the wind. It remains stiff but with the moisture taken out of it.

The great advantage of freeze-drying is that food quality and texture are maintained. Normally the shrinkage and concentration of dehydration forces the various chemical compounds closer together where they may react with each other affecting the flavour and the texture of the food. This does not occur with freeze-drying so the reconstituted food is of a high quality. The only disadvantages are that the process is an expensive one and requires a high degree of technological skill. It has been very successfully applied to meat and fish, particularly shellfish like prawns and shrimps, and it is used to prepare 'instant dinners', notably prawn, chicken and beef curries. Fruit, vegetables and egg have also been successfully freeze dried.

The most popular of all food preservation and storage techniques today, however, is freezing.

Keeping by keeping cold

It is important to realise, although few people do, that the freezing process, whether in factory or home, does not sterilise food by killing off the organisms of disease and decay. Rather it slows down both the activities and reproduction rate of bacteria and the break-down action of enzymes naturally present in the food.

Freezing has a secondary effect, too: by converting water to solid ice crystals it stops many of the chemical changes which can only take place in a watery solution.

Of course, men like the Eskimos have been preserving food by freezing for centuries. In Britain, too, the practicality of, if not the principles behind, preventing food going off by using snow and ice has long been recognised. It is said that the essayist and philosopher Francis Bacon died in 1626 as a result of a chill caught gathering snow with which to stuff and so preserve a chicken. Underground ice houses were common in large country houses in Georgian times, and in the 19th century there was a considerable trade in blocks of natural ice, 'harvested' for example in the New England states and shipped to the Southern States of the USA. (As much as 225,000 tons of natural ice were shipped in the USA in 1872.) In Europe, Norway captured the bulk of the natural ice trade.

By the middle of the century, however, the studies of scientists, such as Rumford, Davy, Joule, Kelvin and others, led to the manufacture of freezing machines. Artificial ice rapidly replaced the natural product: by 1894, a million and a half tons of it were produced in the USA alone.

Better and better freezing machines were developed and by the turn of the century were in widespread use. Not only was food packed in ice to preserve it (and Parisian restaurants were among the first customers for artificial ice) but refrigerated railway cars were also built to transport food. They had ice-packed compartments surrounding the central space where the food was stacked. Ventilators further helped to keep the food cool.

The first problem attacked by the refrigeration pioneers was the preservation and shipping of

71

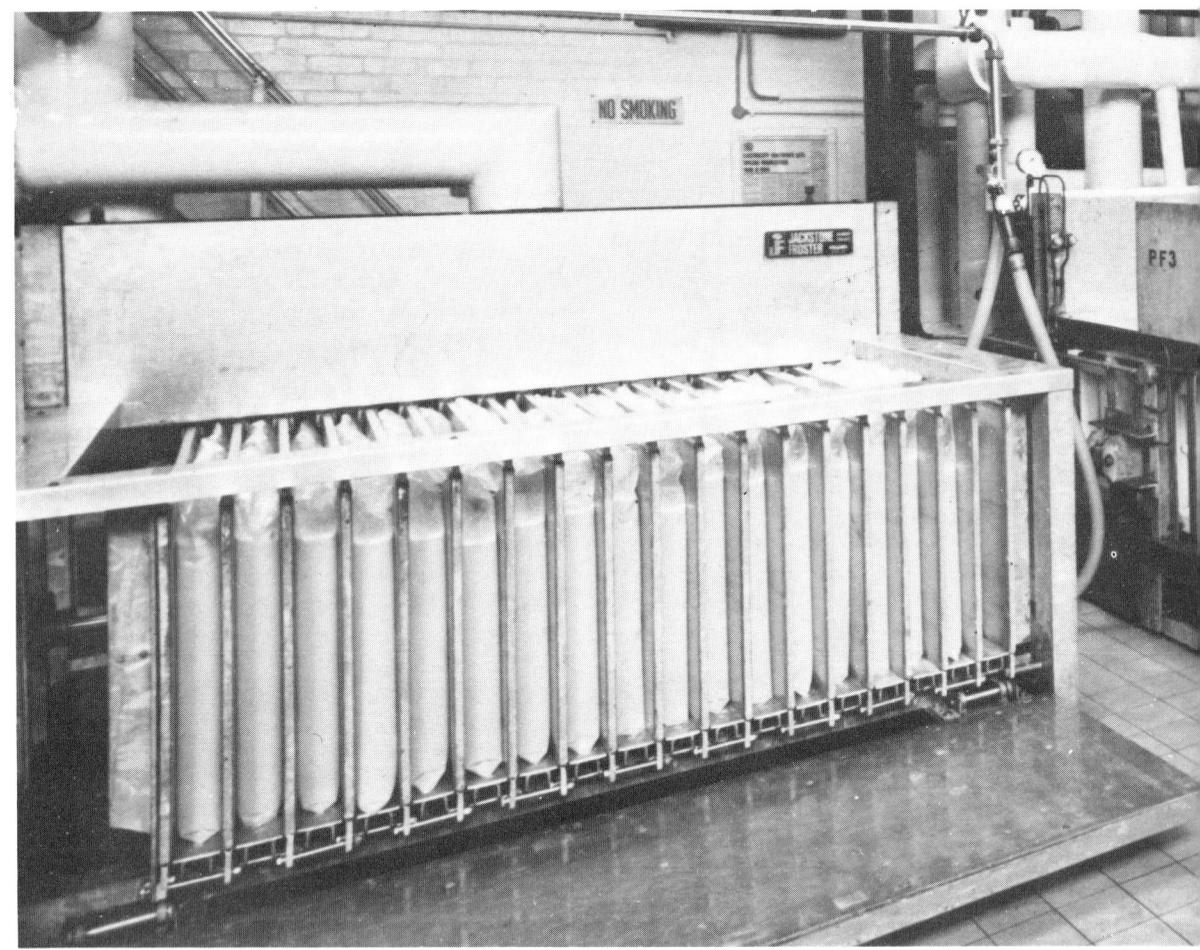

Multiplate freezing.

meat over long distances, notably from Australia and South America to Europe. The meat was not frozen but *chilled*, that is kept at a temperature of about −1°C under which conditions it will keep for about a month.

As we have seen in Chapter Two most foods contain a considerable amount of water and they really freeze solid at about −5°C. If the freezing process takes place slowly, as it does in large meat carcasses, large ice crystals are formed within the cells. They rupture the cell walls and destroy texture. When the food is thawed out it becomes flabby and mushy. At the same time much of the liquid drains away, taking with it nutrient salts, sugars, vitamins and minerals. This not only means a loss in food value but also ruins the food's distinctive taste. In extreme cases it has been

known for thawed food to collapse in a pool of its own juices!

There is, however, a way out of this difficulty. If the food is frozen very rapidly the ice crystals formed within the cells are much smaller and do little or no damage to the texture. Since the cell walls are not broken there is almost no loss of tissue fluids when the food is thawed out.

There are a number of different commercial techniques used in quick-freezing. For fish and meat, the *multi-plate* process is common: the food to be frozen is packed between hollow shelves or plates through which a refrigerant liquid is pumped. The *tunnel* method, used mainly for fruit and vegetables, involves placing a food on a conveyor belt taking it through a current of cold air.

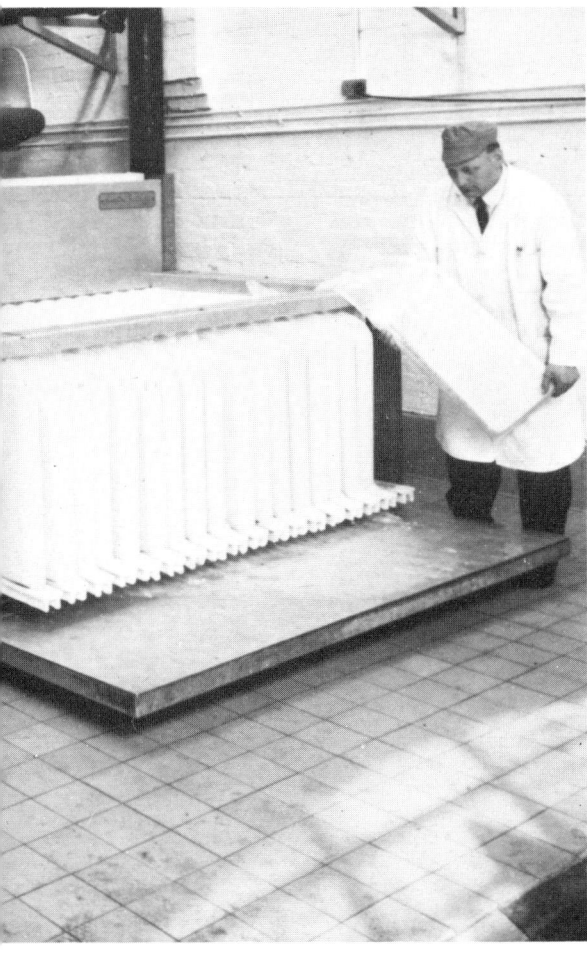

Peas have proved to be one of the foods best suited to freezing and frozen peas are now extraordinarily popular, as the statistic quoted at the beginning of this chapter shows. Another great success story has been in frozen fish. Fresh fish is troublesome to prepare and cook well and it is highly perishable. Quick-frozen battered or breadcrumbed fish portions have, therefore, come like a godsend. Called 'fish sticks' in the USA and 'fish fingers' in Britain, they too have achieved enormous popularity.

The shelves of the domestic refrigerator, now an almost universal household appliance, keep food 'chilled' at temperatures around 5°C. As we have seen, this does not kill organisms but it restricts their growth rate and the food can remain edible for days and even weeks. Temperatures in the freezing compartment are, of course, much lower (around −6°C−−20°C). Most 'fridges now carry a star rating on their freezer compartments: one star means packets of frozen food can be kept for up to a week; two stars means the time may be extended to one month and three stars, to three months.

Once thawed out, *frozen food should never be refrozen*. The microbes burst into activity as soon as the temperature rises and after their chilled dormancy they are much more active in reproduction than normal. So deterioration is rapid. Refreezing merely preserves the larger numbers of organisms and any toxins they may have produced.

Factory food

The magic ingredients in the best food dishes are care and pride: care in the purchase of the finest ingredients and in preparing and cooking them; pride in the skills of culinary art and the presentation of the finished product. The very best chefs – and home cooks too – are those who liberally stir in those ingredients and take time and trouble over food preparation.

When food processing becomes an industry it is far more difficult to instil pride and promote care. Just as a hand-built motor car will inevitably be superior to a production-line model, so too does individually-prepared food always stand a far greater chance of being of better quality. As with any modern factory system, no one worker is involved with the whole of the food process, but is merely a link in the chain, and therefore not

In quick freezing the temperature of the food is lowered to at least −18°C, and frozen food is stored at that temperature.

In a third method, called immersion freezing, the food is plunged directly into a very cold solution. Originally brine was used but recently invert sugar solutions have been tried instead.

Powerful cooling agents like liquid nitrogen have also been used to produce an ultra-rapid freezing action. Strawberries, for example, can be reduced in temperature from 23°C to −12°C in just 30 seconds' immersion.

The greatest advantage of frozen foods is that they are 'convenience foods': the produce is prepared ready for cooking and all the housewife has to do is unpack, unfreeze and cook them. Whole frozen meals are now supplied.

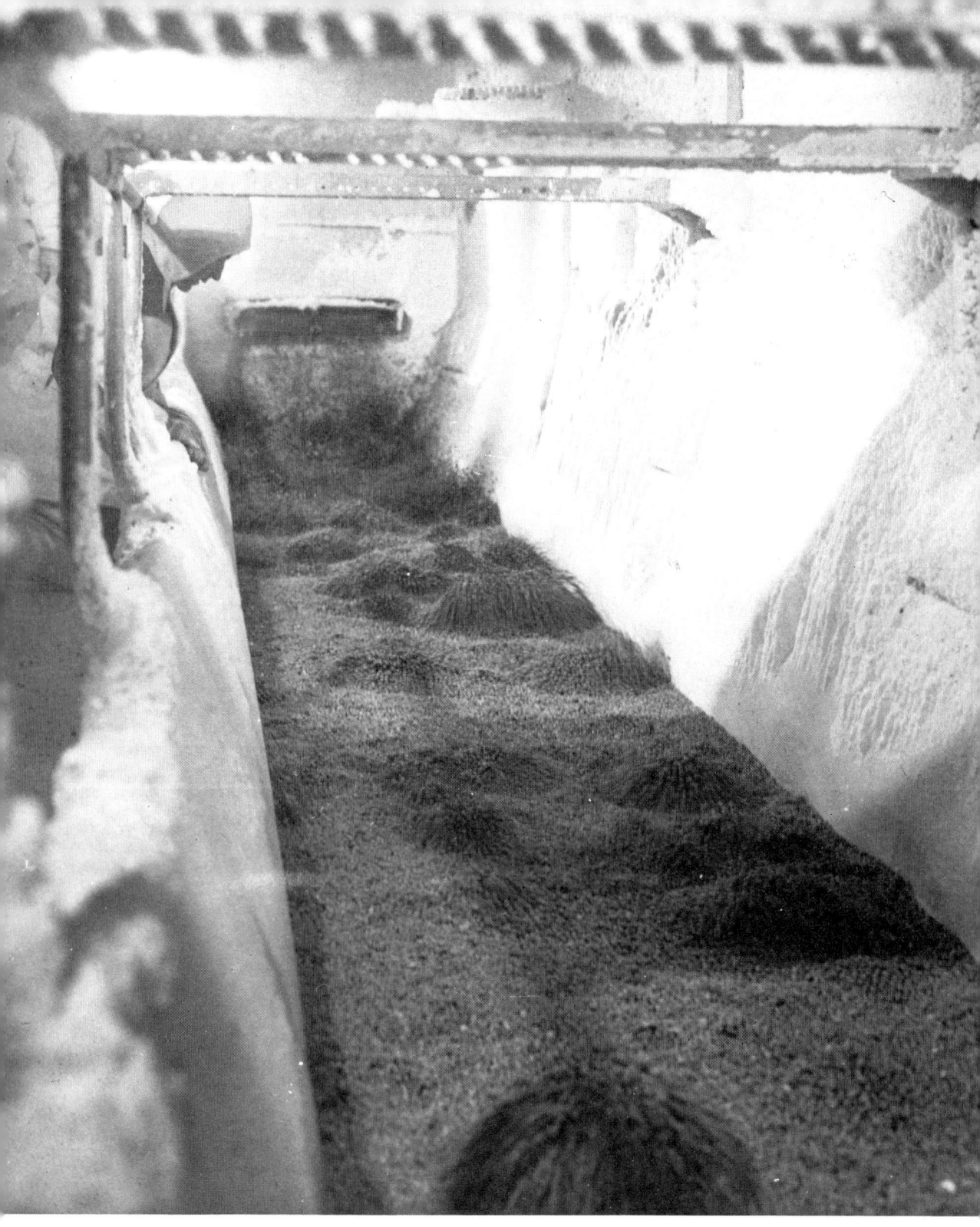

Peas being blown through a freezing-tunnel.

74

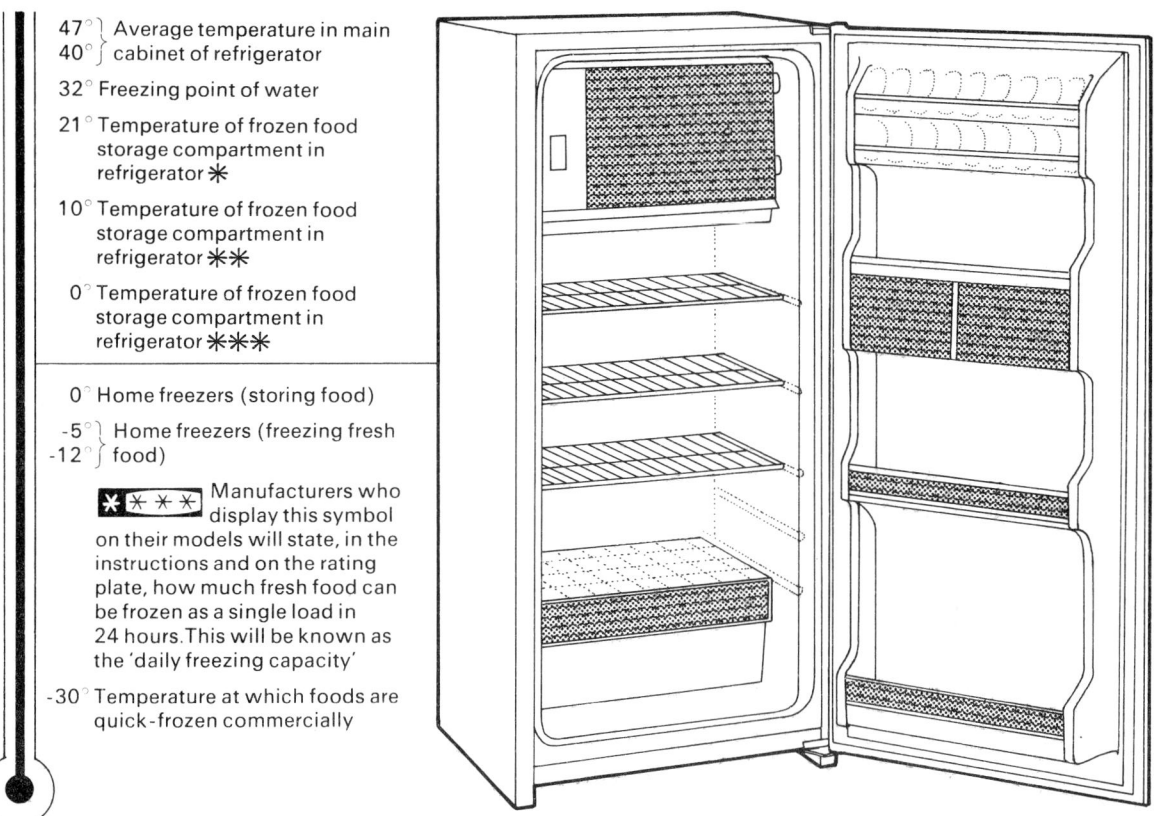

Fahrenheit

47° Average temperature in main
40° cabinet of refrigerator

32° Freezing point of water

21° Temperature of frozen food
storage compartment in
refrigerator ✳

10° Temperature of frozen food
storage compartment in
refrigerator ✳✳

0° Temperature of frozen food
storage compartment in
refrigerator ✳✳✳

0° Home freezers (storing food)

-5° Home freezers (freezing fresh
-12° food)

Manufacturers who
display this symbol
on their models will state, in the
instructions and on the rating
plate, how much fresh food can
be frozen as a single load in
24 hours. This will be known as
the 'daily freezing capacity'

-30° Temperature at which foods are
quick-frozen commercially

Temperatures in different parts of a refrigerator.

intimately involved with the quality of the end result.

Nonetheless, processed food manufacturers start with many advantages. The scale of their operation, for example, means that they can buy in bulk and demand quality raw materials at reasonable prices. They can plan so that they begin their processing when the food, such as fruit or vegetables, is ripe and fresh, and with all the skilled techniques of food technology, they can control their processes with a great deal of accuracy.

But one of the most important considerations, particularly these days, as far as processed food is concerned, is cost. The housewife wants good quality food but she also wants cheap food. The temptation, then, is for the manufacturer to cut costs by cutting corners – buying inferior raw materials for processing and taking less trouble

with the process itself. The result, too often, is a product far inferior to the 'home-made' variety – gristly meat and flaccid pastry in pies, or canned peas that would be better employed as grapeshot rather than on the dinner plate.

The fact remains, though, that the very best processed food can be just as good as, if not better than, a home-produced article. Our choice of manufacturer is still wide and the discerning housewife will soon find which brands to buy and which to avoid.

Economic and other considerations, however, have led to some rather curious ways of doing things in the food industry. Reconstituted chips for instance. It is, apparently, easier to pulverise a potato and then remould it into uniform chip shapes rather than go through the laborious chip-slicing process. You may remember, too, the old-fashioned veal, ham and egg pies with whole hard-boiled eggs embedded in them. Some manufacturers now reconstitute white and yolk and produce a continuous artificial 'hosepipe' of egg of constant diameter to run through the middle. It makes processing simpler but it does remove the excitement of not knowing whether *your* slice is going to have a generous portion of the yolk and white or a mere white sliver from the end of the egg.

Some processed foods, notably processed cheese, bear little resemblance to the traditional product. There is, however, obviously a demand for them and whether we like them or not is simply a matter of taste: we can still pay our money and take our choice.

Mass society and mass catering

Most workers today are unable to get home for their mid-day meal, so industrial catering has become big business too. Almost every large firm in the country has some sort of canteen facilities. Some 75 per cent of such firms organise their own catering, the others use specialised contractors. Again, to save on staffing costs, there is an increasing trend towards convenience foods which merely have to be heated up. Canteen standards vary enormously (that satisfaction is by no means universal can be seen in the evidence that only some 30 per cent of employees on average make use of the canteen for main meals) but the very best can offer a wide choice of hot meals prepared with care and pride.

One of the difficulties of mass catering is trying to ensure that every customer gets a piping hot, freshly-cooked meal. This is next to impossible using traditional catering methods and the food has to be kept warm (usually in metal pans immersed in hot water) for some time before serving.

One new way of overcoming this is 'cook and freeze' where food is prepared in bulk at some central point, the meals arranged in aluminium or paper board dishes and then quick-frozen. They are delivered to canteens in refrigerated vans, stored in cold cabinets and re-heated when needed in forced-air convection ovens. These are very quick: hot meals can be produced within minutes.

Another recent innovation is the microwave oven which can reduce cooking time by as much as 90 to 95 per cent. Some canteens have a system in which measured amounts of the various raw materials are placed on plates and then stored in cold containers until needed. The uncooked meals are displayed in glass-fronted compartments so that the customer can see what he is buying. Coins or tokens put into a slot open the door and with the dish there is usually another token which operates the oven. Within a matter of seconds the customer has a piping hot meal.

Automatic canteens, however, are by their very nature impersonal places and it has to be admitted that there has been customer resistance to their introduction. Gardner-Merchant, the large catering contractors report that out of their 2000 or so operations, only six are automatic vending machines like this. Still, with the high cost of staff – and the difficulty in finding them – there are going to be more and more automated canteens in the future.

Processing, promotion and packaging

Few rational people, I think, would deny that the advantages of food processing techniques such as bottling, canning, drying and freezing outweigh their disadvantages. They enable us to preserve foods from spoilage by microbes, to store them safely and easily at home for use whenever we choose. We can enjoy foods 'out of season' and we can produce quick, tasty and nutritious meals for our families without the time-consuming drudgery so often associated with food preparation in the past. Some processed foods, particularly the frozen ones, can be even fresher than those we buy *au naturel* in the shops. Peas, for instance, are generally frozen within 90 minutes of harvesting while the 'fresh' ones at the greengrocer's may well have taken a week to arrive there.

Nor can there really be objective criticism of the factory preparation of foods to make them more convenient for the housewife to use. Fish 'fingers' and 'steaks', frozen chipped potatoes, sliced beans, ready-made pastry, 'instant' mashed potato – surely these are to be welcomed in an age where more and more women, quite rightly, insist that they are no longer to be chained to the kitchen sink and stove or condemned to a daily shopping expedition. (It might be argued that one of the reasons for the reaction against processed foods is a sense of collective guilt among women because of this very liberation. Generations of conditioning that 'a woman's place is in the home' are not to be cast off overnight. Are the most liberated of women's libbers totally free from a nagging, albeit irrational, sense of guilt? It would be presumptuous for a mere male to analyse the strength of these feelings but one cannot help wondering whether the trend towards lengthy home preparation of exotic and complicated dishes owes something, in part of least, to these considerations.)

Where processed food might justifiably come under fire is in its promotion and packaging. The advertising man in the food industry does not promote his products to assuage hunger but rather seeks to stimulate appetite. As J. Walter Thompson's creative director Jeremy Bullmore has said: 'We sell the myth about food rather than the reality.' Or, as Allan Cameron puts it in *Food – Facts and Fallacies*: 'Manufacturers try to sell an idea rather than a product.'

Cake mixtures, for instance, are usually rather a rather dreary-looking powder so as Cameron says 'the idea is to package it so as to conjure up in the customer's imagination not the reality but an evocative picture of the end product. The packet therefore presents a colour picture of a mouth-watering cake decorated in some exotic way; unfortunately we have now reached the stage where the packet sells the product and – sad thought – we may also have reached the stage where the package costs more than the product!'

This idea-selling can be seen even more strikingly in food advertisements on television, particularly for such products as instant desserts, breakfast cereals and chocolates. The breakfast cereal manufacturers tend to rely on a hearty, out-of-doors, sunshine approach. You, too, can enjoy as healthy and happy a life as those clean-limbed, sun-tanned figures on your screen, simply by opening a packet of cornflakes! A variation is the 'happy home' situation. The family is a joyful, well-integrated unit (do TV advertising families *ever* have a cross word?) and mother and father obviously care greatly about the physical and mental development of their children. One of the principal ways of demonstrating their care and concern, of course, is Bloggs' breakfast cereal.

There is nothing particularly beneficial, from a nutritional point of view, in breakfast cereals. Their main dietary advantage is that they encourage the use of milk, an excellent food for growing children, but on the other hand they encourage the use of sugar too, which has distinct nutritional disadvantages as can be seen in Chapter Five.

More recently it has been the practice to advertise the fact that small amounts of a number of vitamins are added to some cereals. But an ordinary well-balanced diet will provide more than enough of these and there is no need to take in extra supplies at breakfast.

Rather more disturbing is the sales suggestion that a hot breakfast can conquer cold and the image presented of a schoolboy or girl protected by a rosy glow of warmth because mother had prepared some porridgy mixture with hot milk. Although porridge and the like may *feel* warming while you are eating it, it has no significant effect at all on internal body temperature. The burning up of any food – hot *or* cold – produces all the Calories needed to keep the body warm.

The advertising technique often favoured by the chocolate manufacturers is to show the product being enjoyed in exotic or exciting locations by the svelte, the sophisticated and the sexy. The young girl will undoubtedly be prompted to demand a certain brand of chocolate through identification with these high-livers, even if they are bought by a pimply boyfriend at the corner shop, rather than delivered surreptitiously by a black-clad young man with a penchant for jumping on to the roofs of trains or hanging from helicopters.

How you view such promotional techniques probably depends on your attitudes to advertising in general. Mass persuasion certainly helps the development of a consumer society – and provides jobs for the producers. It may also reduce the unit cost of a product by making mass production possible. But it also makes people buy things they do not need. (They may *want* that product but such wants may have been fostered by the advertising rather than because of any intrinsic desire.)

It has been estimated that in Britain we spend some 75 per cent more on food than we *need* to. That does not mean to say that we should all cut down on food consumption – after all, there is far more to life than in providing the bare necessities of shelter, clothing and food. But it does perhaps indicate the need for a little more thought about the reasons behind our buying of some of the manufactured foods.

The difficulties in making a rational choice have been further heightened by the decline of the 'corner shop' and the almost universal introduction of the supermarket. The latter can undoubtedly cut unit costs by high turnover and low profit margins, but the change from the personal service shop, where you have to ask for something, to the self-service store, where you select for yourself, has taken much of the careful premeditation out of food buying.

In fact some surveys have suggested that as many as 70 per cent of self-service purchases are made on impulse and with really expensive items, in elaborate packs, 'impulse purchasing' can account for up to 90 per cent of turnover.

Such issues are legitimate ground for public debate and recent growth in 'consumerism', together with the setting-up of Government-backed organisations, like the Office of Fair Trading, has led to far more investigation and criticism of the techniques involved. Our current concern with the environment, with the enormous amount of waste our society produced, has also turned a critical spotlight on the packaging industry. Few people would wish to turn the clock back to the unhygienic paper bag era, for modern materials undoubtedly keep food cleaner, less liable to damage and often fresher too. It is equally clear, nonetheless, that we really do need to reduce the mass of cellophane, plastics, cardboard and coloured paper that occupies so much space in our weekly shopping baskets.

Such arguments, however, have little intrinsically to do with food processing. If we do not wish to buy factory-processed food we still have the choice not to do so. It may be difficult to resist the blandishments of the advertisements and the beguiling display on the packets, but it can be done. And we members of the public, whether through individual action, through consumer groups or through parliamentary pressure, *can* create our own demand for the food *we* want in the shops, rather than have such a demand thrust upon us.

5 Eating ourselves to death

'They are as sick that surfeit with too much,
as they that starve with nothing.'
  William Shakespeare, 'The Merchant of Venice'.

'More die in the United States of too much food than too little.'
  John Kenneth Galbraith, 'The Affluent Society'.

'The way to a man's heart is through his stomach.'
Fanny Fern, 'Willis Parton'.

'They have digged their grave with their teeth.'
Thomas Adams, 'Works'.

He that despiseth little things — shall perish by little & little

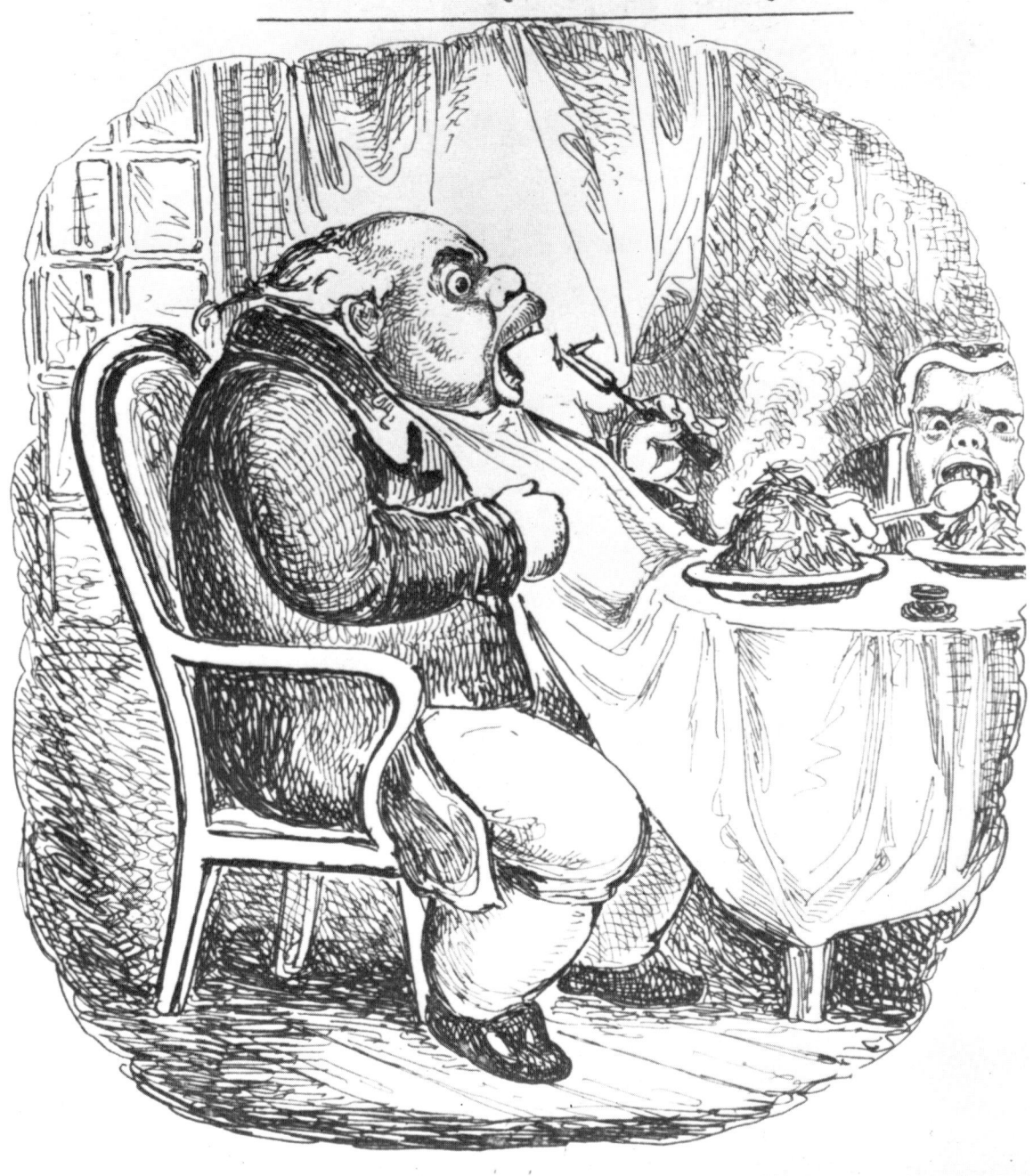

ALDERMEN EATING WIHTE BAIT

Experts in blood fats, implicated as a major cause of heart disease, the greatest single killer in the Western world today, met recently to discuss the value of low fat diets in preventing the disease. After their deliberations they gathered again in the evening for the official conference dinner. This was the menu:

Pâté maison
Poached salmon with hollandaise sauce (made with the finest butter)
Entrecôte Chasseur with french fried potatoes
Soufflé Surprise
Coffee (with cream)

Not exactly the low fat diet preached by many during the day!

Perhaps many delegates ate their meal with equanimity because the role of fats in our diet continues to be a subject for controversy. There certainly seems to be evidence that they can contribute to 'the Western way of death' but so many other inter-related factors are also at work that their precise significance is a matter for continuing fierce debate.

It is a similar story with sugar. The distinguished British nutritionist, Professor John Yudkin, some years ago published a major research paper which seemed to show that the steady increase in sugar consumption was linked in a direct and statistically significant way with the increased incidence of heart and circulatory disorders. Subsequent researchers, however, have cast doubts on Yudkin's findings. As with fats, a large question mark remains.

There is another serious difficulty in coming to a truly objective assessment of the role of diet in disease and that is that food manufacturing has become such big business. It is the saturated fats (see Chapter Two) which are supposed to be the killers, so the manufacturers of polyunsaturated margarines obviously have a vested interest in any research findings which enhance the image of their product and suggest dangers from its rival butter. The sugar manufacturers do not want to see their sales plummet as sweet-toothed consumers switch to artificial substitutes. Any adverse publicity for saccharine or cyclamates is clearly of advantage to them.

So the food manufacturers in these multi-million pound a year industries not only sponsor research, their well-oiled publicity machines are happy to disseminate widely the results of research

work sympathetic to their cause – and their sales – while playing down or ignoring other evidence which may present a contrary view.

In looking at food and health we need to be concerned not just with the potential hazards of specific foods but with the general effects of consumption, or rather, over-consumption. Here the evidence is much more clear cut although finding a solution to the problem is proving extraordinarily difficult.

What is overweight?

The first difficulty in discussing the question of being overweight or downright obese is in defining the terms. Taking the average weights of the population may give us some indication but such averages, which include a large proportion of people who are clearly fatter than they ought to be, provide no precise guidelines to an 'ideal' healthy weight. They can, however, indicate where deviation from the average is positively dangerous as far as our chances of long life are concerned.

One commercial enterprise which has a direct, financial interest in keeping us alive and healthy for as long as possible is life insurance. The later an insurance company has to pay out on our premiums the better, so for many years insurance companies have been collecting data on their clients' weights and attempting to analyse the effects on life span.

A number of different tables have been drawn up, but almost all of them are based on American data gathered over a 20-year period by 26 large life assurance companies and involving nearly five million people. This mass of statistics suggests that men who are 20 per cent above 'normal weight' have a 31 per cent greater mortality rate. It has even been suggested that to be just *10 lbs overweight* carries a *greater health risk* than smoking 25 cigarettes a day.

Such analyses, however, are of necessity based on average weights which are not the 'ideal' or 'desirable' ones. In an attempt to establish such criteria the Metropolitan Life Insurance Company of America produced a table of 'desirable' weights, that is those associated with the lowest mortality. The table, reproduced on page 83, shows these ideals. Weight, obviously, is related to gender (women naturally carry more fat than men), to height and to the size of our frame.

F

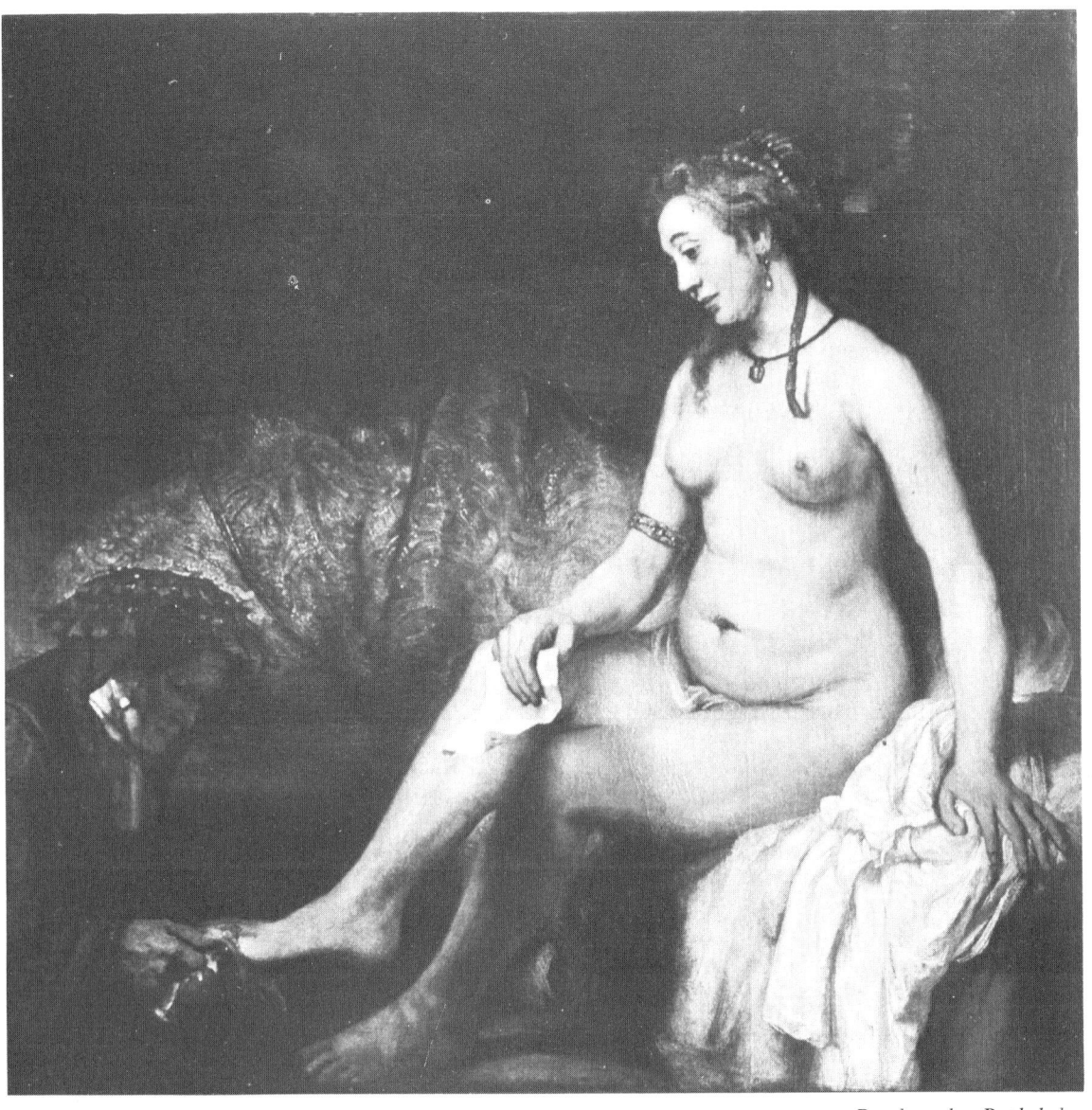

A matter of fashion?   *Rembrandt : Bathsheba.*

The Metropolitan Life table is widely used and generally reckoned to be one of the best available indications of one's best fighting weight. In using it for self-assessment it is important not to cheat by, for example, describing yourself as large-framed when you are really only medium-framed. A good indication is the width of your wrists and ankles and also the breadth of your shoulders. Waist and hip measurements are poor criteria, since it is here that much of the excess fat will have gathered. Nor should a few pounds be added because of advancing age. Certainly the average weight tables do show an increase as people develop into middle-age, but there is no reason why a 50 year old should be fatter than a 25 year old of the same height and build.

Because of the disadvantages of the analyses of average weights, other techniques of measuring obesity have been tried. These include measurements of body fat by underwater

How fat are you?

Life insurance figures show that you have the best health prospects if you are within this range. Weights are measured in indoor clothing and are for people over 25 years of age. 'Frame' refers to your bone structure. For instance, if you have big heavy wrist-bones you can consider yourself as having a large frame.

For men

Height (in shoes)	Small frame Weight in lbs	Medium frame Weight in lbs	Large frame Weight in lbs
5ft 2in.	112–120	118–129	126–141
5 3	115–123	121–133	129–144
5 4	118–126	124–136	132–148
5 5	121–129	127–139	135–152
5 6	124–133	130–143	138–156
5 7	128–137	134–147	142–161
5 8	132–141	138–152	147–166
5 9	136–145	142–156	151–170
5 10	140–150	146–160	155–174
5 11	144–154	150–165	159–179
6 0	148–158	154–170	164–184
6 1	152–162	158–175	168–189
6 2	156–167	162–180	173–194
6 3	160–171	167–185	178–199
6 4	164–175	172–190	182–204

For women

Height (in shoes)	Small frame Weight in lbs	Medium frame Weight in lbs	Large frame Weight in lbs
4ft 10in.	92– 98	96–107	104–119
4 11	94–101	98–110	106–122
5 0	96–104	101–113	109–120
5 1	99–107	104–116	112–128
5 2	102–110	107–119	115–131
5 3	105–113	110–122	118–134
5 4	108–116	113–126	121–138
5 5	111–119	116–130	125–146
5 6	114–123	120–135	129–146
5 7	118–127	124–139	133–150
5 8	122–131	128–143	137–154
5 9	126–135	132–147	141–158
5 10	130–140	136–151	145–163
5 11	134–144	140–155	149–168
6 0	138–148	144–159	153–173

weighing, determination of total body water and indirect calculations based on estimates of lean body mass. Such methods, however, are too complicated to be of general use. Another technique which has gained in popularity recently is measuring the thickness of a fold of skin with calipers. The triceps, at the back of the upper arm, the abdomen and the upper thigh are reckoned to be the best places for taking skinfold readings and there is clearly logic in such assessments for this is a direct measurement of the amount of fat lying beneath the skin. The table (page 84) gives the skinfold thickness regarded as 'representative of optimum nutrition'. Note again that when adulthood is reached there is no reason why skinfold thickness should increase.

The skinfold measurement technique can be used at home. In various areas of the body pinch a fold of flesh between thumb and forefinger. A normal fold should be between half an inch and an inch thick. Anything greater than an inch indicates fatness.

Some doctors believe that we will never be able to define obesity satisfactorily. One expert has written: 'Obesity may be defined as a condition in which the body contours are distorted by a diffuse accumulation of adipose tissue. This depends upon a concept that cannot be defined and which varies with taste and fashion.' And Professor

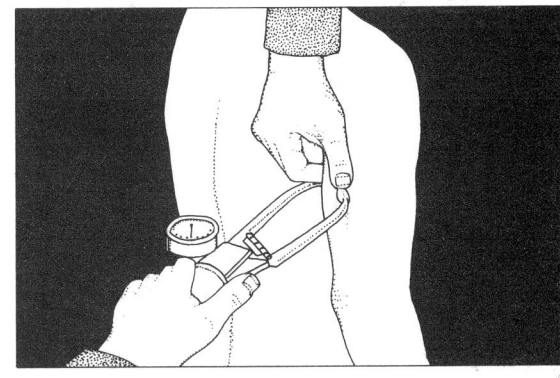

Measuring fat under the skin with calipers.

Skinfold thickness (back of arm) showing
ideal state

Age	Skinfold (mm)	
	Male	Female
1	10·3	10·2
2	10·0	10·1
3	9·3	9·7
4	9·3	10·2
5	9·1	9·4
6	8·2	9·6
7	7·9	9·4
8	7·6	10·1
9	8·2	10·3
10	8·2	10·4
11	8·9	10·6
12	8·5	10·1
13	8·1	10·4
14	7·9	11·3
15	6·3	11·4
Adult	12·5	16·5

Yudkin has suggested that the individual is the
best person to assess whether he is overweight or
not: he can simply look at himself in the mirror or
check whether or not his weight has increased in
the last 20 years or so.

Despite the difficulties in accurate definition the
data from the American insurance companies
clearly showed that a large proportion of the
population has a weight problem: one man in
every five aged 20 or over was at least 10 per cent
above average and one in 20 was 20 per cent
above. Even higher proportions of women were
carrying about too much fat: one in four was 10
per cent above average, and one in nine, 20 per
cent.

There have been no comparable studies in
Britain, but Dr Gaston Pawan, of the Department
of Medicine at the Middlesex Hospital, has
written: 'Nearly half the population of the UK are
overweight and about half of these are frankly
obese.'

Dr Pawan of the Nutrition Society defines
obesity as being 10 per cent or more over the
standard weight/height tables.

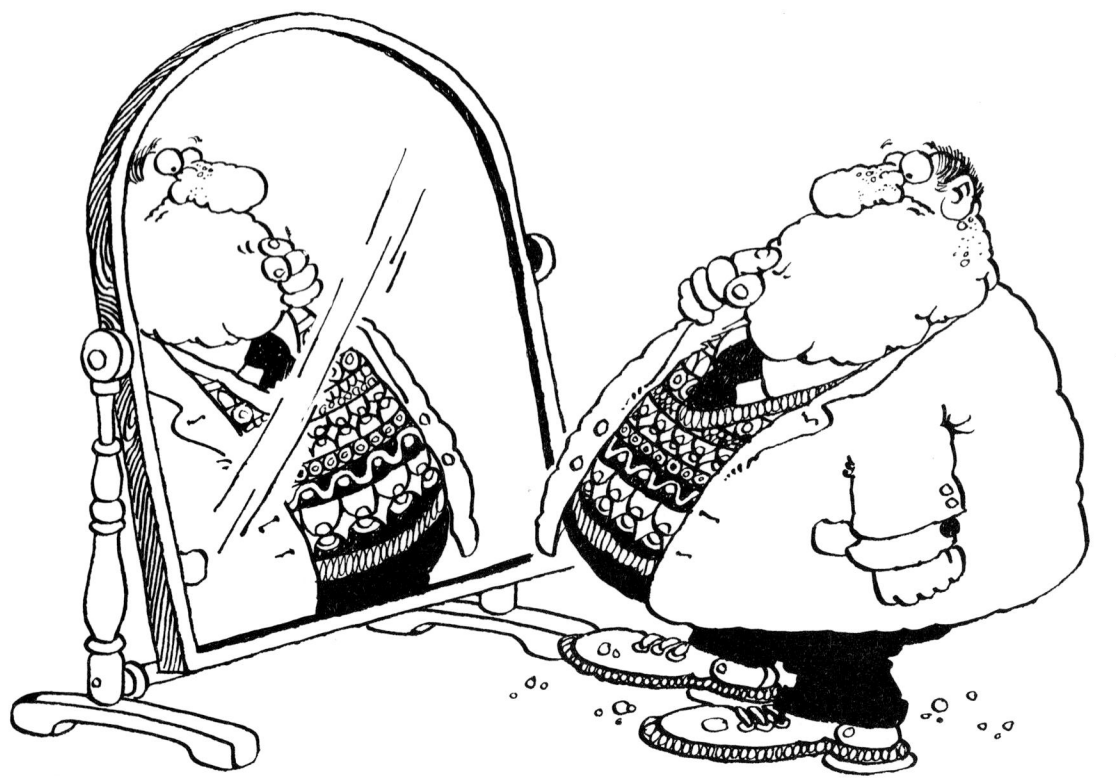

Do we see our bodies as they are?

A study of 2000 business men who underwent a check-up at the Institute of Directors medical centre showed that 19 per cent were between 10 and 20 per cent overweight and that nine per cent were more than 20 per cent overweight.

Whatever the true incidence of obesity it is certain that millions of people are *worried* about their weight. A national survey of 2000 adults found that 13 per cent were currently trying to slim and 25 per cent admitted that within the last year they had made some attempts to reduce weight. Nearly one person in 10 said that within the 12 month period their general practitioners had advised them to slim.

Women seemed far more weight-conscious than men: 35 per cent had tried to slim in the previous year. Of course, many of these attempts were for cosmetic rather than health reasons. The concern was specifically with a reduction in volume rather than a loss of weight for its own sake.

The effects of overweight

Although fashion may dictate much of the current slimming activity it is nonetheless being increasingly recognised that obesity does represent a health hazard.

It is very rare for obesity to be a specific cause of death but it certainly seems to be a significant factor in a number of diseases, although in some the cause and effect relationship is by no means clear cut. There are two factors at work: the increased strain on the body systems simply in having to cope with extra weight and the fundamental effects of fatness on body chemistry and metabolism.

As far as weight is concerned the joints and the ligaments may suffer from mechanical stress, leading to arthritis of the knees and hip, backache and flat feet. Another purely mechanical complication is that a thick layer of fat around the abdomen and trunk obstructs free breathing, so chronic bronchitis in the winter months is often associated with obesity. Hernias, too, are commoner in fat people and they are more likely to suffer from varicose veins. Another less evident factor is that fat people are usually slower in their movements and physical reactions so they are more prone to accident, in the street, at work and at home.

The effects on the metabolism are numerous. The majority of people who contract diabetes mellitus in middle age are obese. The levels of fat-like substances in the blood called *lipids*, the most important of which are *cholesterol* and the *triglycerides*, are significantly raised in the obese. Among the direct effects of this is an increase of stones in the gall-bladder which are composed of cholesterol.

But by far the most significant association between obesity and disease is in the increased incidence of serious heart and circulatory disorders.

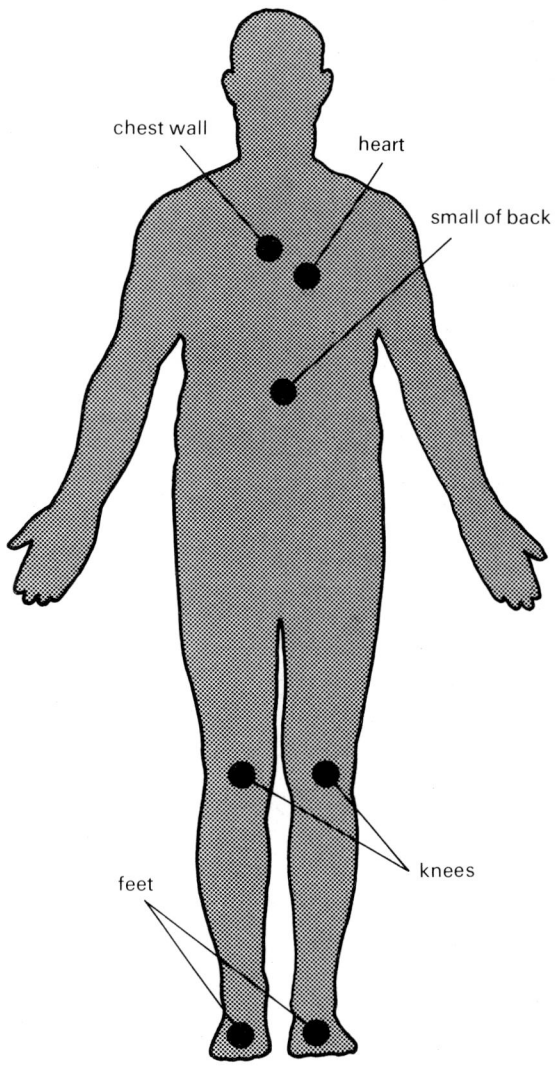

Stress areas in an overweight body.

Clogging the circulatory system

There are a number of causes of heart disease, many of them inter-related but two of the most important are 'hardening of the arteries', technically known as *atherosclerosis*, and high blood pressure or hypertension.

A narrowing and loss of elasticity in the arteries seems to be one of the natural effects of growing old, but atherosclerosis, or excess deposits of greasy material lining the walls of the blood vessels, is statistically linked to increased levels of cholesterol and triglycerides in the blood. And such elevated levels are in turn linked with obesity.

Atherosclerosis not only impairs circulation, it affects the texture of the lining of the arteries which lose their 'duck's back' smoothness. There is a tendency for blood to stick on the blood vessel walls and to form a clot, or thrombosis.

If the clot constricts or blocks blood vessels supplying the heart the result is coronary thrombosis. A blood clot blocking an artery to the brain results in stroke. Deficient blood supply will lead to a loss of the heart's efficiency, leading to a pain in the chest called *angina pectoris*, and to similar losses of efficiency in the brain, the kidneys and the muscles.

High blood pressure aggravates atherosclerosis which in turn can threaten the blood supply to the kidneys. They compensate for decreased supplies by raising the blood pressure, setting up a vicious circle.

Dietary factors affect the heart and circulatory system in other ways too. The fatter you are, the harder your heart has to work anyway to get the blood round the system, and fat people tend to take less exercise than thinner ones, another factor in increasing the tendency to atherosclerosis.

Cholesterol is produced naturally in the body, but the levels are not only affected by obesity and lack of exercise but also by the *type* of foods we eat, specifically by the amount and type of fats consumed.

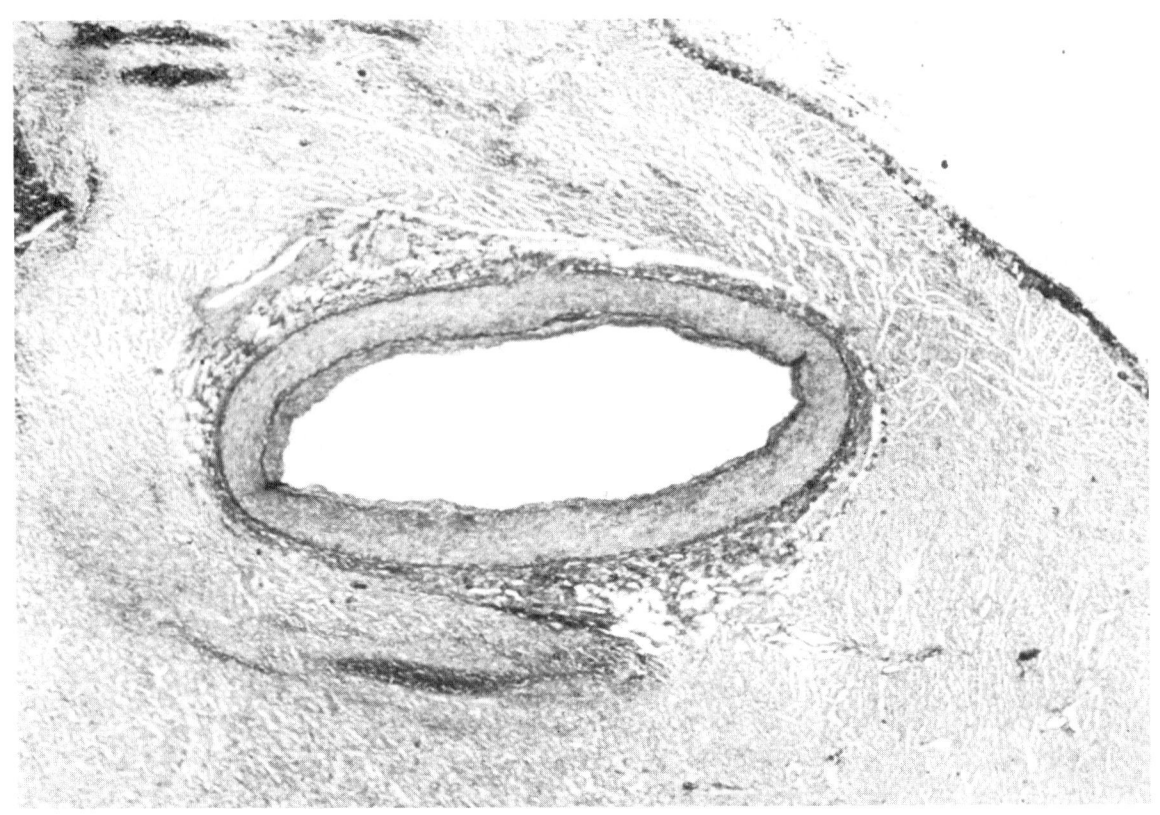

Microscopic view of slice through healthy artery.

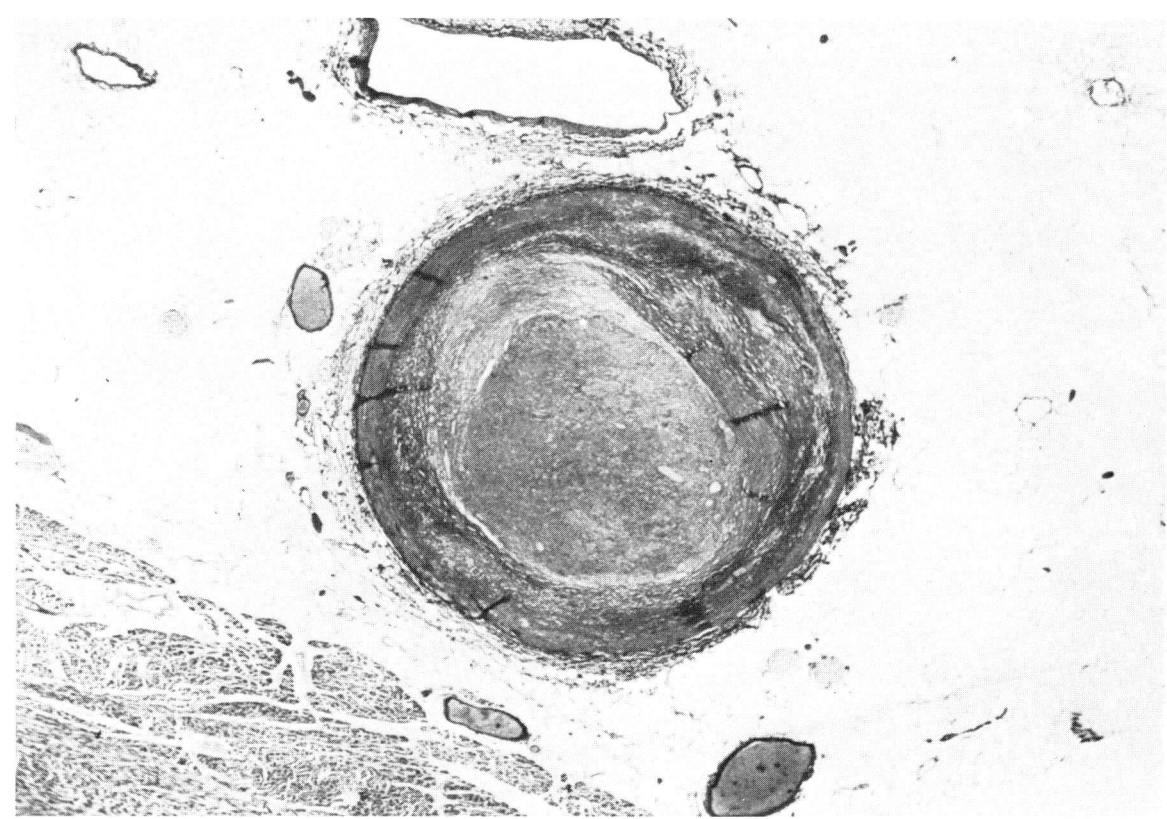

Thrombosis. The artery is totally blocked.

As we saw in Chapter One, fats can be divided into two classes, those made up from saturated fatty acids and those with unsaturated fatty acids. The basic structure of fatty acids is a chain of carbon atoms linked to each other and each linked to two hydrogen atoms. In saturated fatty acids such as stearic acid all the carbon atoms save those at the end of the chain have their full complement of two hydrogen atoms. In unsaturated fatty acids, such as linolenic acid some of the carbon atoms have only one hydrogen atom attached and are linked to each other in double bonds. Fatty acids containing two or more such bonds are known as polyunsaturated.

High levels of saturated fats in the diet are associated with higher levels of cholesterol in the bloodstream. Conversely, the consumption of polyunsaturated fats helps to reduce those levels.

Animal fats tend to contain only small amounts of these protective polyunsaturated fats while vegetable oils and, particularly, fish oils contain much higher amounts.

One of the most significant research projects about the relationship of the different kinds of fat and heart disease was carried out at two mental institutions in Finland. The institutions were chosen because there was a static population available for long-term studies.

The trials lasted the 12 years from 1959 to 1971 and more than 30,000 'person years' of experience was amassed. For the first six years the inmates in one institution were given a diet with an increased proportion of polyunsaturated fats and a corresponding decreased level of saturated fats. This was done by replacing butter and standard margarines with a special soft margarine containing polyunsaturated fatty acids and by skimming the cream off the milk and replacing it with soya bean oil. This mixture is homogenised and is known as 'filled milk'. Inmates at the other institution remained on their normal diet.

Half way through the trials, the positions were reversed, those at the first institution reverting to their normal diets, and those at the second going onto filled milk and polyunsaturated margarine.

The results were impressive. There were only those two differences in diet yet the concentrations of cholesterol in the blood plasma among those in the first institution *rose* from 230 mgs per 100 ml at the end of the first six years to 272 mgs per 100 ml at the end of the second. Conversely the average level at the second institution was 270 mgs per 100 ml and had *dropped* to 235 mg per 100 ml by the end of the trials. It is interesting to note that the level at which *hypercholesterolaemia* – excess cholesterol in the blood – is generally reckoned to begin is 250 mg per 100 ml.

Of greater significance, however, were the analyses of deaths from coronary disease at the two institutions during the survey period.

After adjustments to allow for differences in age during the two six year periods, direct comparison could be made between death rates on saturated and polyunsaturated fat diets. The death rate with the former was 14·08 per 10,000 person-years for men and 7·90 per 10,000 person-years for women. On the polyunsaturated diet, however, the rate was only 6·61 per 10,000 person-years for men and 5·21 for women.

Much has been made of these figures, not least by the manufacturers of a certain brand of polyunsaturated margarine. But it has to be pointed out that, impressive though they are, the results of the Finnish survey by no means prove absolutely that a reduction in saturated fat intake by the general population will lead to a reduction in the incidence of, and deaths from, heart disease. The inmates of Finnish mental institutions obviously lead very different lives from the rest of us. They are less subject to the pressures and pace of 20th century life, for a start, so dietary considerations may well play a much larger role in heart disease among them than it does in the general population.

For the average man – and woman, too, although to a lesser extent – in industrialised society, a bewildering variety of factors may be at work in precipitating heart disease. They include high blood pressure, cigarette smoking, lack of exercise, inherited vulnerability, soft drinking water and a personality which reacts badly to life's everyday stresses and strains. The most telling three factors, however, are high blood pressure, hypercholesterolaemia and smoking.

The relationship between high cholesterol and heart disease has been demonstrated in a number of other surveys. Worthy of mention is the large trial at Framingham, Massachusetts, which showed that the risk of developing *ischaemic* (that is, due to insufficient blood supply) heart disease within an eight year period was five times greater for those 30 to 49 year old men who had begun the trial with the highest serum cholesterol levels.

Earlier evidence had suggested that fat in general was implicated in heart disease, since in populations where fat intake was really low, such as the Bantu tribesmen of Africa and the Japanese, lower levels of heart disease were found. But equally valid relationships exist between heart disease and income, ownership of motor cars and dietary intake of protein.

So there are problems in playing what has been called 'the correlation game'. In an analysis of the causes, costs and treatment of heart disease called 'The Common Illness of Our Time' the Office of Health Economics commented: 'Direct evidence as obtained from a study on 99 bank clerks aged 40 to 55, whose diets were carefully recorded and whose cholesterol was measured, yielded no evidence of any sizeable association between what these men ate and their cholesterol level.

'The study showed a wide range of food intake between the men and also a wide range of cholesterol levels but these were not related to each other. They all had a relatively high consumption of saturated fat and nearly all had a high cholesterol level.

'This suggests that either dietary fat has no direct causal relationship with ischaemic heart disease or that it is only below a certain level of fat intake that there is a direct relationship with mean cholesterol levels and ischaemic heart disease; above this level of fat intake no simple effect on cholesterol level is exerted and it is suggested that this level obtains in many Western communities including the United States and Britain.'

Even reducing the cholesterol, by diet or with drugs, of those with naturally high levels 'may not necessarily reduce their risk of coronary artery disease' says the OHE report. It adds, however, that 'it is nevertheless true that any over-eating can lead to obesity with general higher rates of sickness and perhaps of heart disease.'

Nonetheless in the United States, where heart disease kills some two-thirds of a million people a year, great emphasis has been placed on the role of diet. In 1972, for example, The Food and

Nutrition Board of the National Research Council and the American Medical Association recommended a partial replacement of the dietary sources of saturated fat with sources of unsaturated fat and also prescribed a reduction in cholesterol-rich foods.

Increasing attention has been focused recently on other fats in the blood called the triglycerides (because each molecule of fat contains three fatty-acid units). Studies at the University of Uppsala and the Karolinska Hospital in Sweden suggested that people with higher cholesterol levels only ran a two to three times higher risk of ischaemic heart disease than those with normal levels. If cholesterol was normal, but triglycerides raised, the heart disease risk was $2\frac{1}{2}$ to $3\frac{1}{2}$ times normal, and if both were raised the risk was increased fourfold. Reduction of cholesterol without a corresponding reduction in triglycerides still left people highly vulnerable to heart disease.

Raised triglyceride levels *(hypertriglycerid-aemia)* are usually easier to correct through diet and drugs than high cholesterol levels, the Swedish researchers told a World Health Organisation conference in 1972. It is also intriguing to note that while cholesterol patterns are very similar for males and females from 20 to 50 years old, women – with a lower incidence of heart disease – have lower triglyceride levels.

As with cholesterol, much more work needs to be done before a definitive answer can be given about the role of fats in our diet. The current evidence does seem to suggest that we do eat more fat than is good for us. It has been calculated that the minimum amount of fat needed to make our food palatable is that which provides about 20 per cent of the diet's total energy value. But wealthy people – both in the West and the East – eat in such a way that fats contribute around twice as much as that. An earlier American recommendation (in 1968), this time from the National Academy of Sciences, advised middle-aged men that they could best avoid a coronary by restricting fat intake to 25 per cent of the diet's energy value. Yet the average levels in the USA are 42 per cent and in Britain we still obtain well over a third of our energy from fats.

There are a number of diets designed both to cut down the total amount of fat in the diet, to switch a significant proportion of the intake from the saturated to the unsaturated and polyunsaturated varieties and to reduce cholesterol

Which fats raise your blood-cholesterol?

These raise the level	These have little effect	These lower the level
Butter	Peanut oil	Maize (corn) oil
Margarine	Olive oil	Cottonseed oil
Beef fat		Sunflower seed oil
Mutton fat		Soya bean oil
Cooking fat		Sesame oil
Lard		Safflower oil
Coconut oil		Fish oils

High-Cholesterol foods

Type of Food	Cholesterol mg per 100g ($3\frac{1}{2}$ oz)
Dairy Produce:	
Egg Yolk	1,500
Whole egg	550
Butter	250
(cp. milk	11)
Meat:	
Brains	2,000 at least
Kidney	375
Liver	300
Sweetbreads	250
(cp. chicken	60)
Fish:	
Roe	300 or more
Oysters	200 or more
Lobster	200
(cp. fish fillets	70)

blood levels. The tables show the cholesterol and fat contents of some common foods, although it must be emphasised that blood levels are not directly related to food levels. It can be seen that brains, egg yolk and offal such as kidney, liver and sweetbreads have high concentrations, as do roe and oysters. Margarine made purely from vegetable fat and cereals, on the other hand, have no cholesterol in them at all. In fact, cholesterol only occurs in foods of animal origin.

As far as the fats are concerned, a switch from animal fats such as butter and lard to vegetable and marine fats and oils will increase the intake of unsaturated fatty acids. Changes in dietary intake are not too difficult since some 40 per cent of our fat comes from butter, margarine, cooking fats and oils and these can be switched to unsaturated substitutes with ease.

One curious footnote about fats is worth mentioning. Although the trend today is towards soft and polyunsaturated margarines, initially the manufacturers wanted to make their product

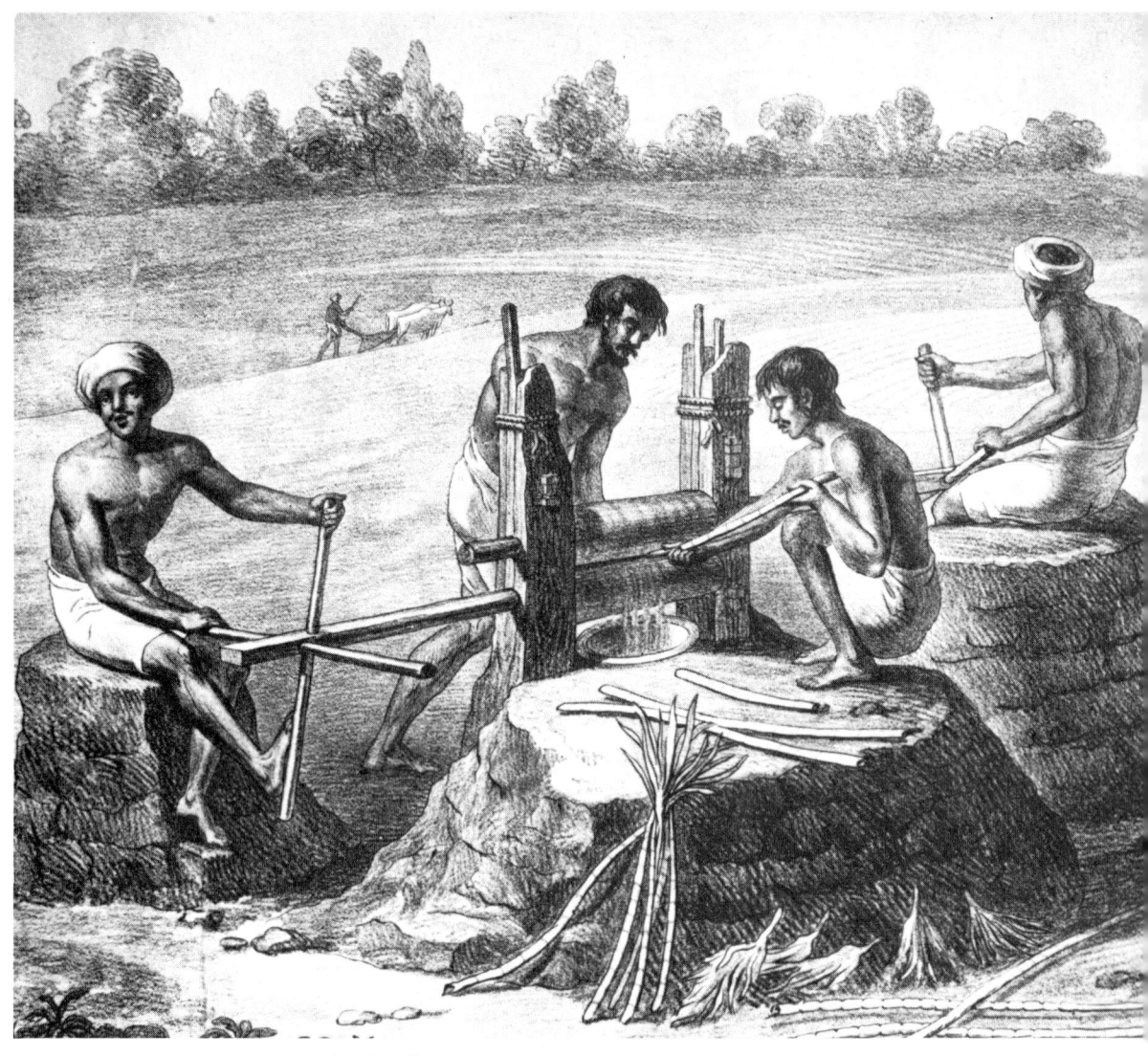

Indians crushing sugarcane in a hand mill.

'hard', of the same consistency of its arch-rival, butter. And the way they did that was to convert chemically unsaturated vegetable oils into the saturated type!

It was noted earlier that by no means all experts are convinced that dietary fats and cholesterol play a really significant role in heart disease. One leading researcher in Britain, Dr Malcolm Carruthers, has written in his book *The Western Way of Death*: 'Cholesterol was the ideal choice of culprit as it had been found on the scene of the crime by microscopists. Its footprints in the shape of characteristic clefts could clearly be seen in the walls of some affected arteries, where it could be stained a spectacular and guilt-ridden red colour. The chemists were also happy to testify to cholesterol being the 'bad egg'. There was plenty of it to measure, both in the blood and in the food, and the levels of the two tended to bear a suspicious, albeit inconstant relationship.

'Being nice and stable both in and out of the body, and not one of these will-o'-the-wisp compounds whose blood levels vary widely during the day and disappear as soon as you think you've

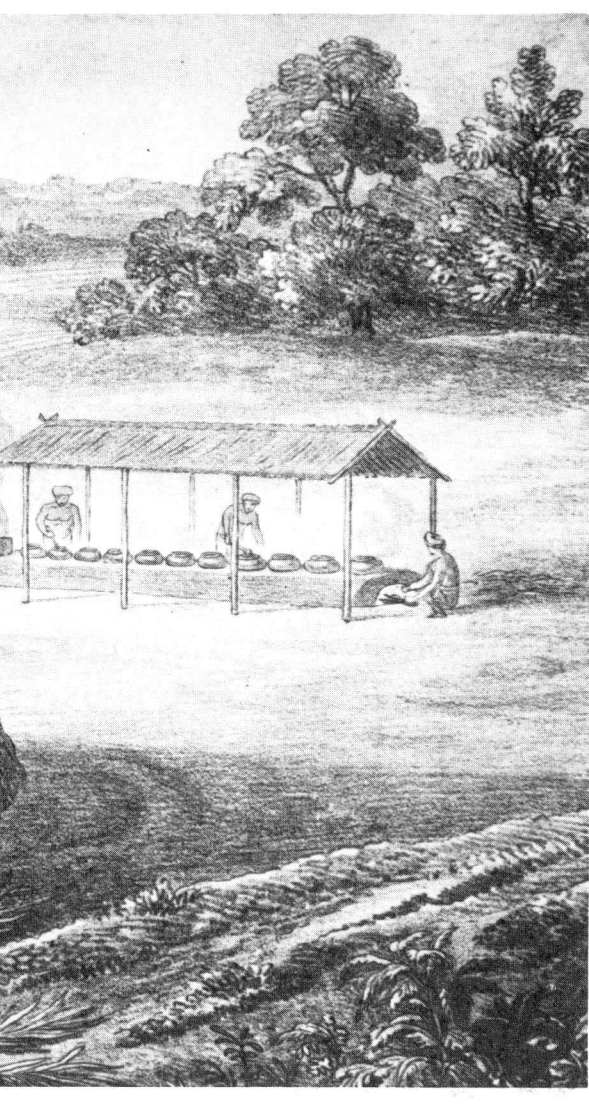

coronary circulation. Heart attack rates obstinately continued to rise.'

It should be pointed out that Dr Carruthers (who incidentally unearthed that heart disease conference menu given at the beginning of this chapter) is mainly interested in the role of emotional and physical stress in the disease. Nonetheless, his view of the significance of diet is clear: in his 132 page book he devotes less than a page and a half specifically to diet.

While the cholesterol/triglyceride/saturated fat debate continues, a new dimension in the diet and heart disease story was added a few years ago by Professor John Yudkin. His hypothesis was that at the root of the problem was not the saturated fats at all but that widely-used product sucrose – ordinary sugar.

The sugar saga

A hundred years ago the average person in Britain probably ate little more than five pounds of sugar in a whole year. Today every man, woman and child consumes an average of 105 pounds of it annually, or the best part of two pounds each week. In fact Britain has the dubious distinction of being among the most sweet-toothed nations of the world. We take in those weekly two pounds not just in the sugar we stir into our tea and coffee, or sprinkle on our breakfast cereals but in a bewildering wide variety of manufactured foods. Chocolate, ice-cream, confectionery, cakes and jams are obvious examples. But sugar can be found in large quantities in many other products as well. Another look at the list of contents of the packets, cans and bottles on your kitchen shelves will show you just how ubiquitous a product it is. It is even added to items such as tomato soup and tinned meat.

It is rather difficult today to contemplate a sugarless world but prior to the end of the 18th century it was the prerogative only of the rich. And while today we are prepared to pay a premium for brown sugar, then the insistence was for white, the whiter the better – and more expensive. We may suppose that man has always had a sweet tooth and he would have satisfied this from the earliest times by eating fruits, berries and honey. Our liking for sweet things is demonstrated in the analogies we use in everyday speech. We talk of 'the sweet life', La *Dolce* Vita and the charms of Irma la *Douce*. We may whisper sweet

got them trapped in a test tube, it was a sitting duck for the collection of chemically incriminating evidence. From here it was a brief exercise in *ad hoc* reasoning to the "It's what you eat that does it" school of thought that holds sway to this day.'

Saturated fats, says Dr Carruthers, later joined cholesterol among the 'baddies' so that (and he exaggerates somewhat!): 'The market soon became saturated with unsaturated food products. This was good for the circulation of grocery products and magazines with complicated diet sheets, but appeared to have little effect on the nothing to our sweethearts or call them honey and sugar.

Yet we do not *need* to eat sugar. It is merely a carbohydrate source of energy and could easily be replaced by any other energy-giving food: carbohydrate, fat or even protein. True, it is useful in giving structure to some foods, such as jam, biscuits or cakes but pure sugar is a source of what the nutritionists call '*empty calories*'. There is energy there and nothing else; eating a slice of bread for its carbohydrate content, on the other hand, would give you some protein, vitamins and minerals as well.

So sugar may 'dilute' the diet. One tends to replace some of the other carbohydrate foods with the sugar and thus cut down on the intake of their associated proteins and other nutrients. There's little doubt, too, that a craving for sweet things does lead people to eat more than they really need, leading eventually to obesity and its attendant problems.

But just what is that sweet substance – refined sugar – so many millions crave?

The art of sugar refining is thousands of years old and techniques are described in some of the earliest records from India and China. The basic process is to extract sucrose (a double sugar composed of glucose and fructose. See Chapter Two) from sugar canes. These were crushed between heavy stone rollers to extract the juice or syrup. This was then boiled to a sufficient concentration to form sugar crystals as it cooled. Unfortunately the first crystals to form are not pure sucrose, but a mixture of sugar and various dark-brown pigmentations.

It seems that it was the ingenious Arabs who developed the first refining process to produce purer and whiter sugar. They crystallised the sugar in conical moulds forming an inverted dunce's cap, with a hole at the pointed end through which the liquor drained away. Then a mixture of clay and water was poured in and

Antigua: windmill for cane-crushing on a plantation.

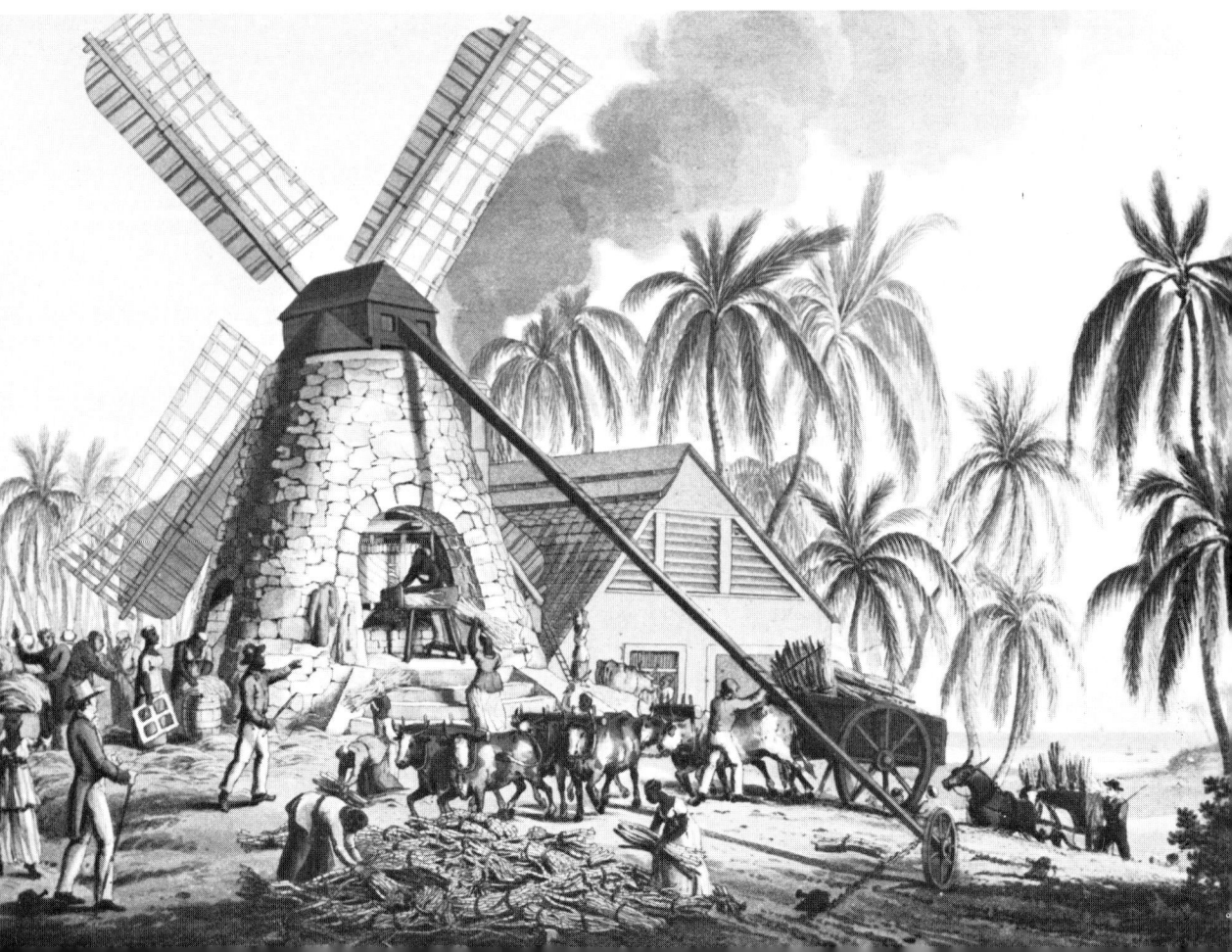

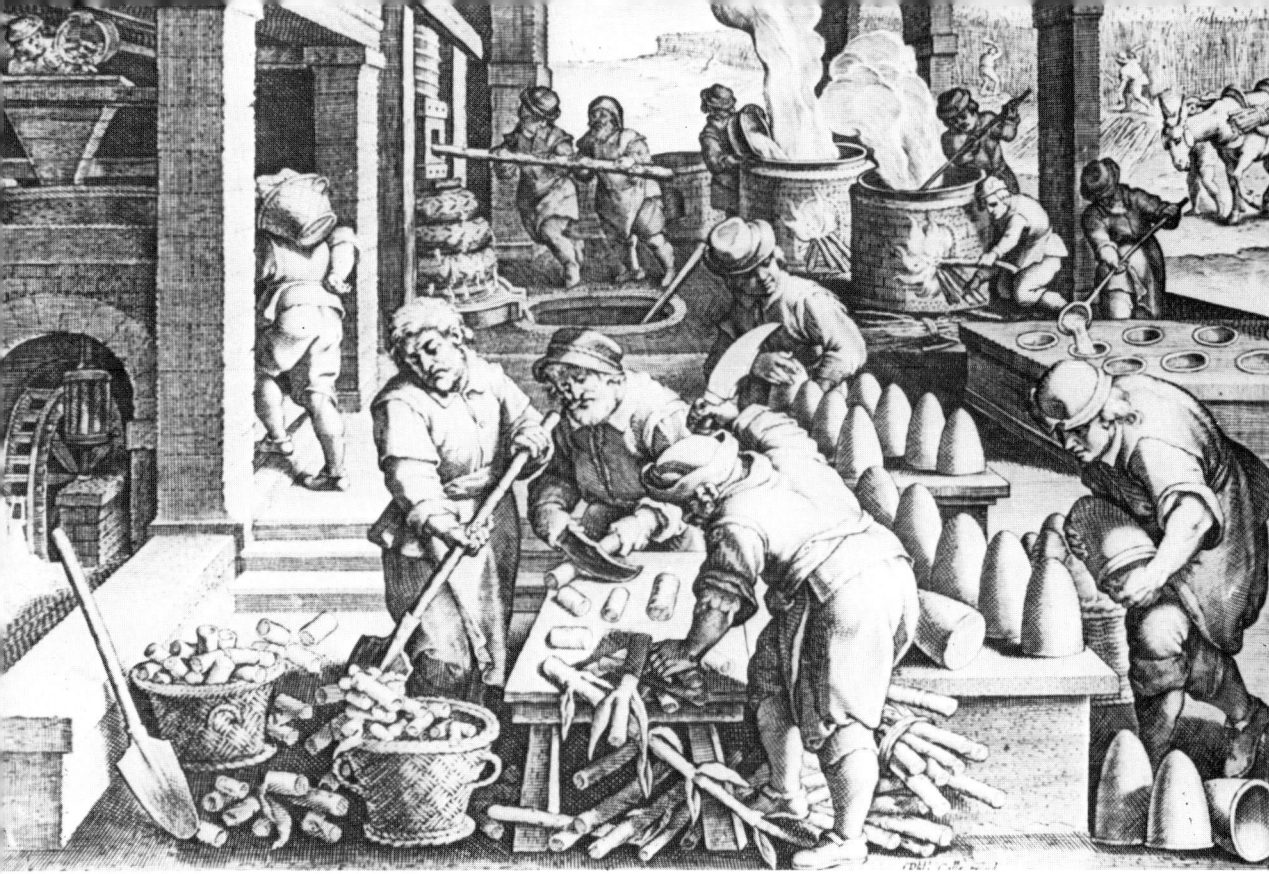

Refining sugar, 17th Century. Cones are visible.

allowed slowly to percolate through the impure crystals. The molasses sticks to the clay and gradually drains away with it. The process, known as 'claying' was repeated until pure white crystals remained. These were compressed into sugar loaves. Imports to Britain began in the middle of the 12th century but it was not until the beginning of the 13th that significant quantities were coming in, from Venice. Today's housewife, grumbling at rising sugar prices, may care to note that the cost then was equivalent, in today's terms, to some £25 a pound.

Modern techniques are considerably more sophisticated and extraction processes considerably more powerful. Crushed sugar cane, for example, is milled under steel rollers which exert pressures of 200 to 500 tons to extract every last drop of juice. This is sieved, has lime added to neutralise organic acids, boiled, decanted and concentrated to a syrup before being allowed to cool and crystallise. The *mother liquor*, or molasses is separated from the unrefined sugar by high-speed spinning in a centrifuge.

Refining now involves mixing the raw sugar crystals with a thick syrup, adding lime and bubbling through carbon dioxide which causes waxes, gums and other impurities to form a sediment which can be filtered off. The syrupy mixture is then finally purified by passing it through finely-ground *bone char* (made by charring small pieces of animal bone to form a porous substance composed of calcium phosphate with a layer of charcoal).

The syrup is then boiled in vacuum pans until it crystallises – the size of the crystals can be determined at this stage. The refined sugar is then washed, dried, sifted and packed. Sugar beet, which supplies about one-third of the world's sugar needs (or rather *demands*) has only been used for a century or so. The refining process is identical and so is the end product. The only difference is that the sugar is washed out of the beet with hot water rather than squeezed out.

Refined sugar is one of the purest of all manufactured foods, being some 99.9 per cent sucrose. Far from being pleased with such purity,

93

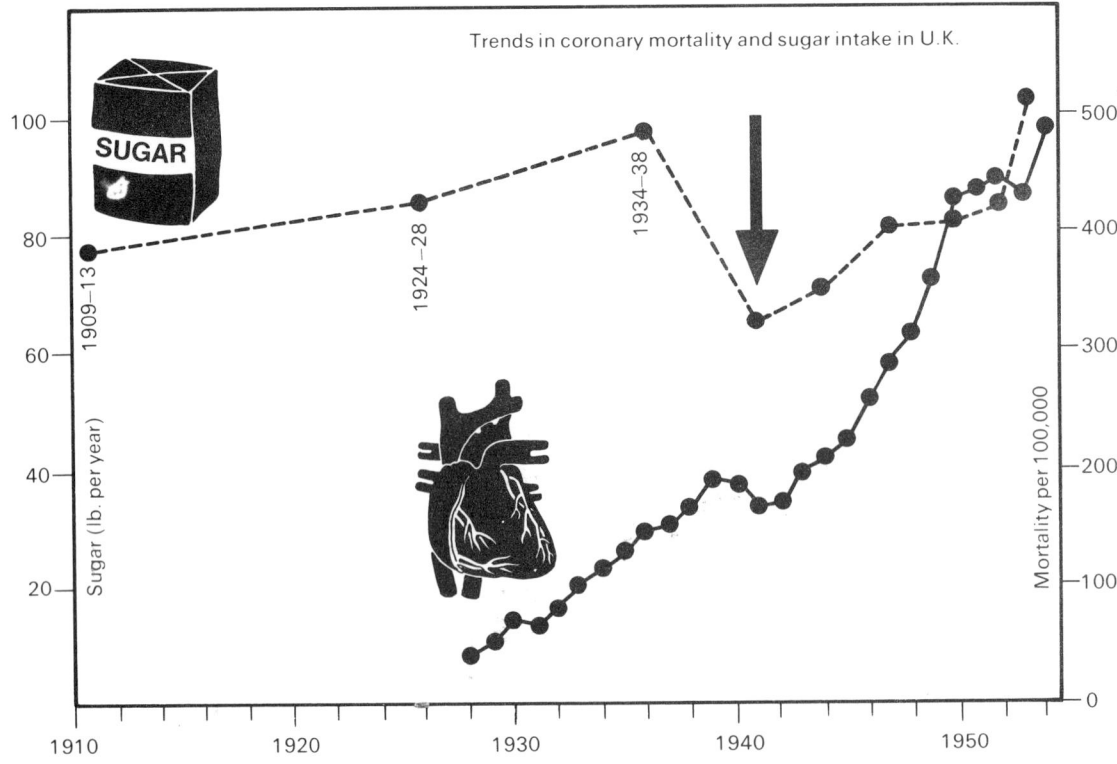

Graph suggesting a relationship between sugar intake and heart disease.

some condemn such sugar for being merely a 'chemical' and that somehow the 'goodness' is lost. But if you want sugar as an energy source, it is the sucrose you are after.

The hypothetical sugar/heart disease link is largely based on a number of studies correlating the increasing though fluctuating incidence of the disease with similar flunctuating increases in sugar consumption. But there is a biochemical rationale for proposing such links.

When sugars – or carbohydrates that yield sucrose and fructose on digestion – are eaten, it leads, not unnaturally, to an increase in blood sugar. There is an increase, too, in the levels of blood *fats* which seems reasonable since carbohydrates are easily converted to fat. What has been established recently, however, is that the level of these fatty substances is related not only to the amount of carbohydrate eaten, but to the type of carbohydrate as well.

Animal experiments have shown that sugar and carbohydrates containing *sucrose* and fructose (fruit sugar) lead to higher levels of blood cholesterol and triglycerides than those containing *starch* and glucose. And the animal experience, in such species as rats, rabbits and baboons, can, it seems, be translated to man too.

In one trial, for example, one group of men were given a low fat, high sucrose diet and compared with a similar group on low fat, high starch diets. Blood fats were measured over a 25 day period, during which levels rose in the first group and declined in the second. Assessing the situation another way round, another team of researchers questioned men admitted to hospital with heart disease about their dietary habits. It was found that their sugar consumption was nearly twice as high as the 'controls', a comparable group of healthy men.

On the other hand, an official Medical Research Council investigation into the sugar hypothesis failed to find any significant connection between sugar consumption and heart attacks. MRC investigators at four centres, two in London and in Edinburgh and Glasgow, studied the records of 150 men who had had heart attacks and slightly more who had not. The heart attack victims *had* slightly more sugar in their blood than the others but the differences between the two groups were so small that they could have been attributable simply to chance. The MRC researchers suggested that the real culprit was probably smoking, since smokers generally have a sweeter tooth than non-smokers.

Nonetheless there is a considerable file of statistical evidence to bolster the suggestion of a sugar consumption/heart disease link. American negroes, for example, have a high incidence of heart disease whereas African negroes, with similar racial characteristics run a considerably lower risk. The sugar consumption in Africa is only six pounds per person per year while the average American negro eats some 80 pounds of it every year. Similarly, the Indians who live in Natal, and consume some 110 pounds of sugar annually have a much higher incidence of heart disease than their racial brothers at home in India who eat only 12 pounds annually.

In some countries too we can find strong correlations between the graphs of mounting sugar consumption and the escalating incidence of heart disease: Czechoslovakia is a good example. But in Britain, as the graph shows, the correlations are far from perfect. In the 1930s both sugar consumption and the death rate from coronaries rose, and at the beginning of the Second World War, they dropped together. But between 1940 and 1950 the death rate from coronaries doubled while sugar consumption remained lower than before the war.

So we are still left with an enormous question mark over the precise role of diet in heart disease. It clearly makes sense in the treatment of those who have already suffered heart complaints to reduce the levels of cholesterol and triglycerides circulating in their blood. But medical opinion is divided on the necessity of recommending major dietary changes in the rest of the apparently healthy population.

With so many other factors involved, dietary change alone would be unlikely to produce any dramatic reduction in the coronary death rate. To do this we must seek ways of changing our whole life style, of which diet is just a part.

Setting up the rot: sugar and tooth decay

While some sugar and disease doubts remain, there is one condition which has reached truly epidemic proportions, in which sugar has been conclusively shown to be the principal villain. Tooth decay is rampant and few, if any, of us escape it: 99 per cent of Britons and 95 per cent of Americans are estimated to have dental caries. More than one-third of all adults in Britain have *no natural teeth at all* and some 25 per cent of our five year olds will be wearing dentures of one sort or another by the time they are 20!

Our teeth are composed of a stout shell of bone-like material called *dentine* protected by an outer layer of an even harder and denser material called *enamel*. Hard as it is, enamel is susceptible to attack by a variety of bacteria and in particular by the acids they form in conjunction with sugars.

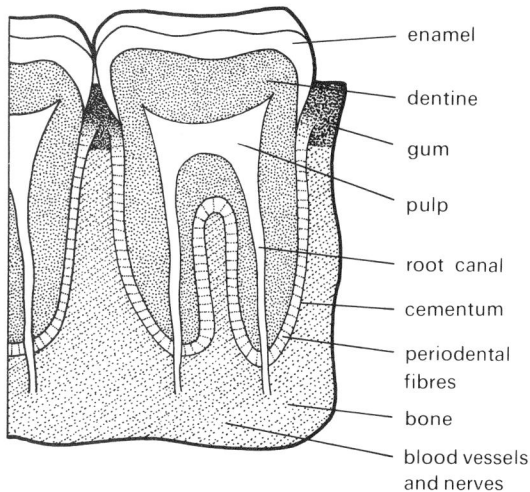

enamel

dentine

gum

pulp

root canal

cementum

periodental fibres

bone

blood vessels and nerves

Clean teeth have no sticky plaque, protecting bacteria.

At the root of the problem is a nasty, almost transparent substance called dental *plaque* which is continually being deposited on the surface of the teeth. It is composed mainly of bacteria, together with saliva and tiny particles of debris from food and from the cells of the gums which have died and been replaced.

Sticky carbohydrates, particularly a polysaccharide called *dextran*, help to keep the plaque firmly gummed to the tooth. When carbohydrates, and above all, sugars, come into contact with the plaque they form acids which attack the surface of the enamel and form a small crevice. This in turn enables the plaque to penetrate further into the tooth and the acids produced to extend and enlarge the hole.

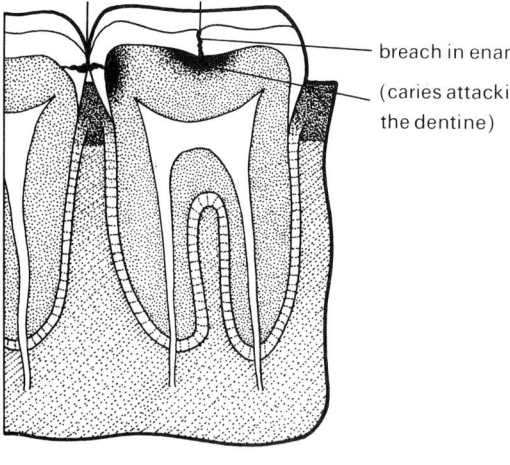

Plaque helping bacterial attack

breach in enamel
(caries attacking the dentine)

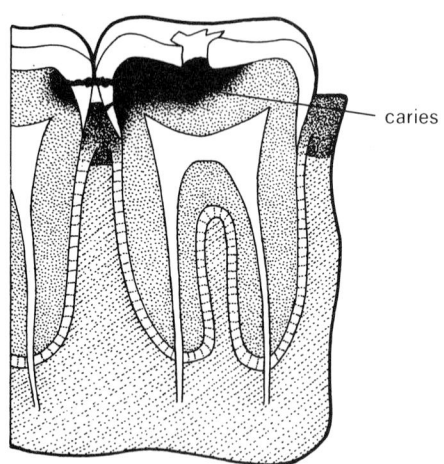

caries

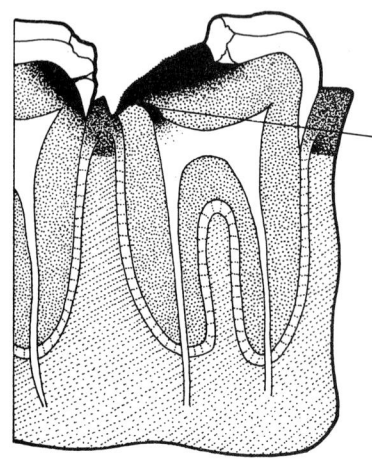

collapse of enamel, exposure of pulp and nerve

Stages in tooth decay.

The most harmful bacteria multiply best without oxygen. At first tiny particles of food between the teeth help to protect them from the air. As they get deeper into the airless crevice, however, they are able to multiply even faster. Once a hole is well established other types of bacteria can attack the pulp, the soft tissue in the interior of the tooth. When these become inflamed the nerve endings within are affected, and toothache sets in.

Sucrose, that is cane or beet sugar, produces dental decay much more rapidly than other carbohydrates or even other sugars like glucose or lactose. The reason seems to be that certain mouth bacteria have a remarkable capacity to convert the relatively simple sucrose rapidly into the large complex and sticky carbohydrate, dextran, which keeps the plaque firmly attached to the tooth's surface.

The texture of the food we eat is important in this context, too. Cooked starchy foods are sticky and also help the plaque to adhere to the teeth. Fruit and vegetables, on the other hand, have a fibrous structure and help to keep the mouth clean mechanically by rubbing against the teeth and so preventing a build-up of debris. So such foods as celery and carrots, which require determined chewing, will help prevent decay. Chocolates, boiled sweets, sticky cakes and ice cream can all help to promote it.

Mind you, in talking about diet and dental decay the experts have by no means been consistent. It is not so long ago that the British Dental Association was talking about the apple as 'nature's toothbrush' and suggesting that while an apple a day might not keep the doctor away it would certainly help to keep the dentist at bay.

Food and teeth

Good for teeth	Bad for teeth
Eaten after *other food*	*Particularly* between *meals*
Raw carrot	Sweets
Celery	Confectionery
Raw cabbage	Soft drinks
	And maybe
Apples!	*Cheese!*
Some experts now think the sugar in apples may do more harm than good	Recent research suggests that cheese eaten *last* at mealtimes may actually protect teeth from plaque

Now they are having second thoughts because, after all, there is a fair amount of sugar in an eating apple. BDA Secretary, Robert MacLean, said recently: 'An apple is better than nothing for cleaning the teeth after a meal but it cannot be used instead of a proper cleaning with a toothbrush, especially last thing at night.'

One simple solution to the dental decay epidemic is in our own hands: it's called a toothbrush. The sad fact is that most people cannot be bothered to clean their teeth properly. Actually the phrase 'cleaning the teeth' is misleading since it is cleaning out the gaps between the teeth which is of paramount importance, not shining up the enamel. Six-monthly visits to the dentist are essential too. He can help directly by scraping away the line of *tartar* which often forms at the point where teeth and gums meet. This tartar not only promotes decay by providing shelter for the plaque bacteria but also leads to gum inflammation and gum disease, which is as big a problem as tooth decay. Fluoridation of the water supplies helps prevent caries in children by promoting the growth of stronger, more acid-resistant teeth, but regular cleaning is still as essential as ever. The ultimate answer may well lie in the development of vaccines, which are at present undergoing clinical trials. They are made from the enzymes of one of the mouth bacteria. These enzymes are responsible for promoting the change of sucrose into sticky dextran. Injections of the vaccine produce antibodies which prevent the bacteria from producing the harmful enzymes. The result: no plaque, no acid and no decay. It is going to be several years, however, before they are fully tested and in general use.

To sum up the overall effects of diet and disease we can say that there are both doubts and certainties. It is certain that the obese are far more prone to a wide range of diseases than the slim. And it is certain that sucrose is the prime culprit in tooth decay. While there are strong indications that fats, particularly of the saturated variety, and possibly sugar too, increase the risk of heart disease, the doubts, for the present, remain.

Nonetheless, it makes sense for all of us to look more closely at what we eat. Much of our fat, carbohydrate and sugar intake in the over-fed Western world is at best unnecessary and at worst, potentially hazardous. But we do not need to become food faddists in order to eat more sensibly. Nor are crash diets to reduce weight the answer: the likelihood is that after a few weeks of misery we will be back to our bad old ways. Rather we must seek techniques of incorporating enjoyable but healthy eating habits into our total way of life.

G

6 Of bread, bran and health food

'Give us this day our daily bread . . .'

The Lord's Prayer.

'Many diseases of Western civilisation have appeared only in the last century. We believe that they owe their origin, at least in part, to the removal of indigestible fibre from the carbohydrate foods that constitute the major part of our diet.'

Dr Denis Burkitt et al, 'Journal of the American Medical Association', August 1974.

'Vegetarianism is harmless enough, although it is apt to fill a man with wind and self-righteousness.'

Robert Hutchinson.

'When Mr Denis Burkitt, the distinguished Medical Research Council scientist eats a meal aboard an aircraft, fellow passengers often stare when they see him pull out a little bag of coarse, powdery brown substance from his flight bag and sprinkle it on his food.'

So began a report in the medical magazine *Interface* on one of the latest developments in what seems to have been an almost perpetual argument over the role of one of the most basic ingredients in our diets – the cereals.

What Denis Burkitt was doing was sprinkling *bran* on his food, to give his digestive system some fibre to work on, some 'roughage' conspicuously absent from the pre-packed convenience foods invariably served up by the world's airlines.

Burkitt, affectionately known in medical circles as 'The Bran Man', and a growing number of other experts, believe that bran may well give us protection against a wide range of conditions, from varicose veins to diverticulitis (inflammation within the large intestine), from appendicitis to coronary thrombosis and even cancer of the colon. It is even suggested that fibre may react with bacteria in the gut to protect us from the toxic agents and prevent unwanted side effects from some of today's powerful drugs.

The products of cereal crops, like bran and flour, are such fundamental foods that it is not surprising that they have been the subject of discussion and argument for hundreds of years. It is bread in particular that has raised the greatest controversy, unabated to this day. So before looking in detail at the claims now put forward for one cereal product, bran, let us first look at the whole vexed question of the preparation of cereals for, and the baking of, 'the staff of life'.

Is white bread a nasty, noxious unhealthy product, adulterated with unwanted chemicals and cooked to render it nutritionally meaningless? Is brown bread the only wholesome product from the bakers? Why has there been so much controversy?

Much more than a food

Bread is so universal a food and so much a part of everyday life that it has become much more than merely something we eat, and has often taken on a magical and mystical symbolism. The Arabic word for bread actually means 'life' and the Christian church, in the communion service, uses it as a symbol for the Body of Christ, as a spiritual food. The Egyptians, the Jews, the Greeks, all attached great religious significance to bread. In many cultures and communities magical properties were vested in the loaf specially baked from the last sheaf of wheat harvested in a field. It was supposed to protect all who ate it from misfortune and ill-health.

The 'neolithic revolution', in which man gradually changed from being primarily a hunter and gatherer to a more settled farming and stock-breeding existence, took place, it now seems, at more or less the same time in various parts of the world, around 10,000 years ago. The changing weather conditions, as the glaciers of the last Ice Age receded, promoted the growth of wild cereals which in turn encouraged the formation of permanent settlements. It was not long before man learned that it was better not to harvest all the grain, but leave some seeds behind for next year's crop and from this it was but a short step to sow the seed evenly by hand. The early cereals were primitive forms of wheat and barley, with a rather loose ear, as shown in the picture. Through generations of cultivation and selection of the best the ear became shorter and more compact.

Of course, the second problem was to select the edible part of the grain from the outer sheathing of tough material, the chaff, by no means a simple task. It was soon discovered that the separation was made much easier if the ears were slightly toasted and threshing was often carried out in pits floored with heated stones. Even so further processing was necessary, and the grain was rubbed by hand or between stones to remove all the chaff (and some of the bran, the thin tough coat round the seed).

But raw grain is indigestible to man. The nutritionally valuable wheat germ (see diagram) is embedded in a starchy mass, the *endosperm*. Surrounding this is a closely-packed layer of protein granules – the *aleurone layer* – and then the bran. For the grain to be digestible it must be cooked but there is considerable doubt as to the earliest methods. Many prehistorians favour the pit-boiling technique. Reay Tannahill describes it in her book *Food in History*: 'A pit or depression in the earth was first lined with flat, overlapping stones, to prevent seepage, and then filled with water. The water was brought to the boil by heating other stones or pebbles directly in the hearthfire and manhandling them (by some

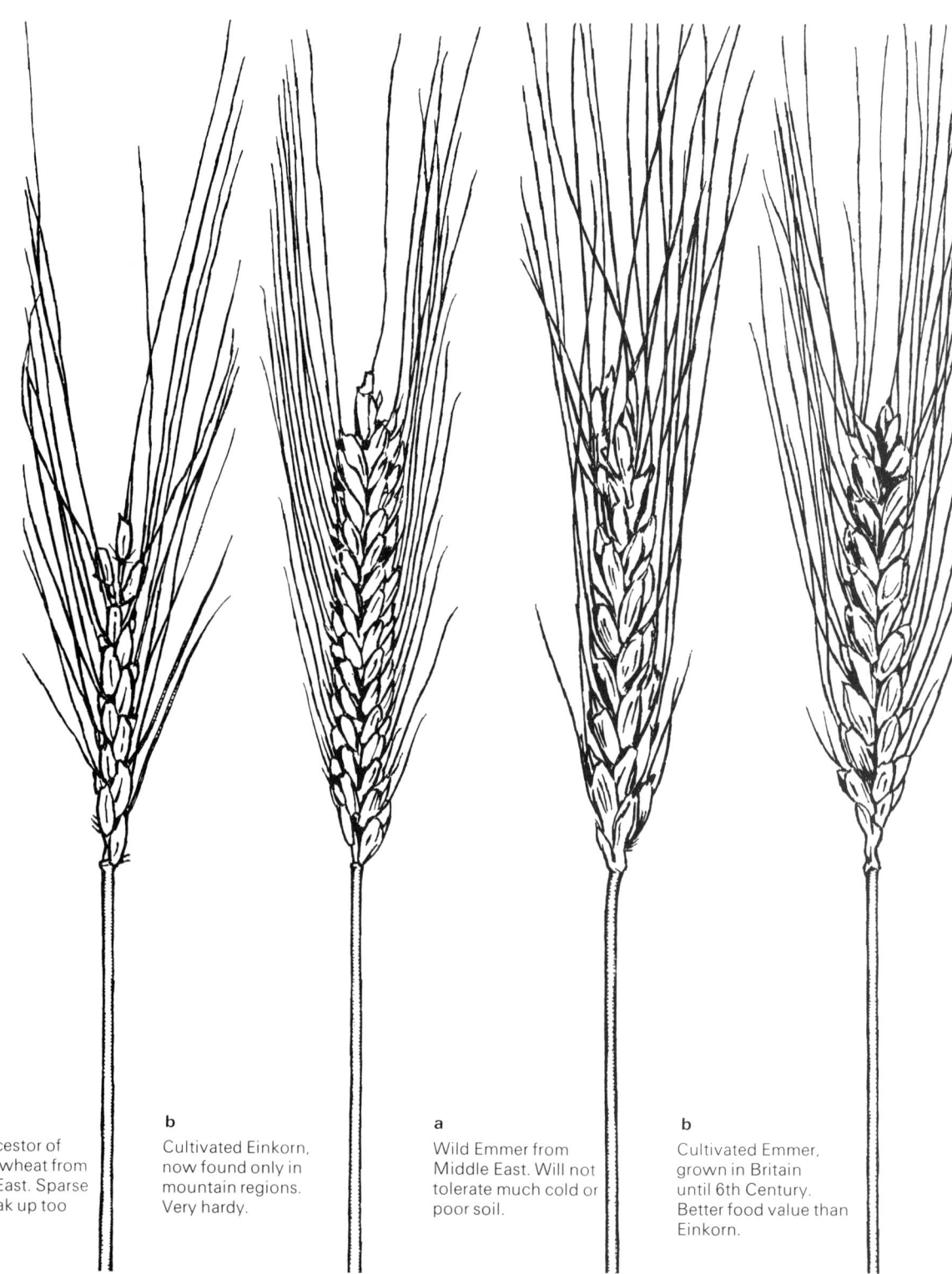

a

Wild ancestor of
Einkorn wheat from
Middle East. Sparse
ears break up too
easily.

b

Cultivated Einkorn,
now found only in
mountain regions.
Very hardy.

a

Wild Emmer from
Middle East. Will not
tolerate much cold or
poor soil.

b

Cultivated Emmer,
grown in Britain
until 6th Century.
Better food value than
Einkorn.

Wild ancestors and cultivated forms of early wheat.

unspecified means) into the water. While the food was cooking more hot stones were added to keep the water at a suitable temperature.' But as she adds: 'Even by neolithic standards, pit-boiling must have been irksome and inconvenient, especially if it came as a climax to the exacting process of rubbing and pounding.'

Leavened and unleavened

What seems much more likely is that the first cooking process came about by accident while the grain was being heated to break up the chaff. Heat regulation, after all, was very haphazard and it was inevitable that some of the grain became thoroughly roasted through, if not charred. When such grain was cleaned and pounded in a mortar the resulting *groats* would be digestible but rather too dry to eat, and the next logical step would be to mix it with water to make a doughy paste.

This, it has been pointed out, would be very similar in taste to the Greek *maza* and the Roman *puls*, grain pastes which formed a major part of the diet in classical times. It is not difficult to imagine, either, the subsequent discovery of the merits of heating a flattened portion of stiff grain paste on a firestone to create delicious, crusty, hot unleavened bread. Add a little fat or salt and, according to the grain used, you have produced something little different from the modern Scottish oatcake, Indian chapati or Mexican tortilla.

The trouble with such breads, however, is that while they are tasty hot they become leathery and indigestible when cold. And, unlike grain paste they will not keep for long. It was not for some time – probably around 1000 BC – that the solution was to be found, in *leavened* bread. The word leaven comes from the Latin *levare* to raise, and from the same source, *levis* is Latin for light. It requires a particular kind of wheat, which can be threshed without heat. Other cereals like barley or millet are unacceptable because of their chemical composition and rye, which may be used, was not known in the civilised world before the first pre-Christian millennium.

The key to the leavening process, of course, is yeast which, in the right conditions, breaks down sugars in the wheat grain's starchy endosperm to form bubbles of carbon dioxide gas, causing the dough to rise and giving it a spongy texture. If the grain has been heated before the yeast is added, leavening cannot occur. But heat afterwards sets the bread in its new open texture.

Egypt is generally credited with the discovery of raised or leavened bread and doubtless it was entirely accidental, some leavening yeasts fortuitously drifting into wheat dough left ready for baking. It was clear some sort of fermentation process was at work so known ferments were soon added artificially – wine juice was popular and the Gauls were known to have used the foam from the top of their home-brewed beer. It was possible, too, to mix the wheat flour into a kind of porridge and wait until it went sour. As Pliny the Elder commented: 'Manifestly it is natural for sourness to make the dough ferment.'

It is not necessary, however, to start afresh with each baking since a little dough left over from a previous batch may be added to the next as a 'starter'. Although today dried yeasts are available the best bread still comes from that in which the leavening process is begun by such a 'sour dough starter'.

The advantages of leavened bread – its superior texture and better keeping properties – did not mean that it instantly replaced the old flatbreads or grain pastes. Indeed right up to the Middle Ages it was uncommon in Northern Europe.

A question of colour

We have noted earlier that there is far more to any food than merely its nutritive value, its taste or its texture. With bread, the one aspect that has raised more controversy than any other is colour. Until comparatively recently the clamour was always for white bread, the whiter the better. For hundreds of years, the miller and the baker strove to meet the public demand. You could judge a man's status as much by the colour of his bread as by the cut of his cloth. And as our towns grew in the late 18th and early 19th century, so too did the calls for a whiter loaf steadily increase.

As soon as technology was able to give the people what they wanted and techniques had been developed for producing really cheap flour for white bread, we saw the beginnings of a remarkable *volte face* in public attitudes to bread and the colour question. There are certainly tens of thousands, and possibly millions, who feel today that white bread is at worst a poison and at best nutritionally inferior. Brown, they say, is beautiful and one popular writer has gone as far as to say: 'There can be no shadow of doubt . . . that every time a housewife buys a loaf of white bread for her family she is taking an unnecessary risk with their health.'

The writings of modern nutritionists on the comparative merits of breads of different colours have an air almost of desperation: the objective facts are straightforward enough but bread raises such subjective passions that they realise that informed argument alone will never convince those who hold contrary views. In *Food – Facts and Fallacies*, Allan Cameron concedes that 'bread is such a common food, eaten by nearly everyone nearly every day, that we all count ourselves experts on the subject.' He adds: 'Unfortunately we are only experts on the trivialities and being without the necessary facts and knowledge, we substitute emotion and conviction. This results in generating a great deal of heat without throwing much light on the problem; it also results in different people holding opposite convictions with the utmost tenacity, even though neither conviction is upheld by an appraisal of the facts.'

Magnus Pyke, in *Food and Society*, acknowledges that even those with 'knowledge and facts' fall short of objectivity: 'Few people are able to discuss the composition of bread temperately, and this intemperance is often shared by those who use scientific information in their arguments.

'The danger of a little scientific learning about bread is not that people are likely to poison themselves by reaching a wrong conclusion, or even to affect their health to any marginal degree. It is, rather, that confusion and error are always to be deprecated, and a student of nutrition who holds with violence to an untenable position about bread on allegedly scientific evidence is more likely to reach an equally unfounded conclusion on other matters of more importance.'

So it is not without a little trepidation that we embark on an attempt to present fairly the nutritional facts about brown and white bread.

Modern milling

The essential differences between white bread and brown result from the way in which the grain is milled, or ground to a flour. In essence, the greater the efficiency in grinding down the interior starchy part of the wheat, the endosperm,

and discarding the other parts of the grain, the whiter the finished product.

Of course the tendency for the unscrupulous to by-pass the tedious and costly paths to excellence by cheap and rapid processes which give the public a semblance of what they want is by no means a modern phenomenon. It is well over 150 years since the first 'white bread scandal' hit the headlines.

Even the best quality flour has a yellowish tinge when freshly milled and it needed to be stored for several months both to improve its colour and to enhance its bread-making properties. The short cut was to add alum, chalk or ammonium carbonate. And in pursuit of profit bakers were soon adulterating their flours with careless abandon.

In 1820 Frederick Accum, a German-born chemist living in London, set about them – and other food adulterers – in his book *A Treatise on Adulteration of Food, and Culinary Poisons*. The bakers were not Accum's only target: he revealed that pickles owed their tempting green colour to copper, that the rind of Gloucester cheese was frequently given its rich orange hue by the addition of red lead, and that 'crusted old port' was often nothing more than new port with an artificial crust of supertartrate of potash.

On bread, Accum wrote: 'This is one of the sophistications of the articles of food most commonly practised in this metropolis, where the goodness of bread is estimated entirely by its whiteness. It is therefore usual to add a certain quantity of alum to the dough; this improves the look of the bread very much, and renders it whiter and firmer. Good, white and porous bread may certainly be manufactured from good wheaten flour alone; but to produce the degree of whiteness rendered indispensable by the caprice of the consumers of London, it is necessary (unless the very best flour is employed) that the dough should be bleached; and no substance has hitherto been found to answer this purpose better than alum.'

The storm raised by Accum's book was so strong that he was forced to leave the country and, after the initial excitement had died down, little or nothing was done for the next 30 years. It was not until the 1850s that a long series of articles on food adulteration was published in the authoritative medical journal *The Lancet*. In one *Lancet* investigation 49 loaves from various sources were analysed: not one was free from alum. *The Lancet* exposés led directly to the passing of Britain's first Food and Drugs Act in 1860. This Act was considerably revised and toughened in 1872.

Fortunately for the bakers new, and legal, methods of producing good white bread flour were becoming available through the development of new milling techniques, especially the superseding of mill-stones with steel rollers. The reason why stone ground flour is brown is that it is 'wholemeal', that is it contains all the parts of the grain: the bran, the aleurone grain layer and the germ, as well as the endosperm. Fine bran particles darken the flour, and the fat and enzymes mean that it does not keep so well.

The steel rolling processes can produce a fine flour which is almost entirely endosperm, and when these techniques were introduced it was soon possible to produce a white flour that was cheaper than wholemeal flour. White bread was no longer a status symbol.

It was not long before there was a backlash and protagonists of brown bread berated the nation for eating white. Prominent among there were the Reverend Sylvester Graham and a Dr T. R. Allinson. Graham propounded a lengthy argument which concluded that since God had put all the parts of the grain together it was harmful, if not sinful, to separate them: what God has joined together let no man cast asunder. And harking back to the 'Good Old Days', he declared that the strong men of the past had eaten only coarse wheaten bread to preserve them in the strength of their limbs. Dr Allinson combined, in Magnus Pyke's words 'a vehement advocacy of brown loaves with teetotalism and anti-vaccinationism as well'. Allinson held that 'persons who eat white bread often suffer from an inward craving or sinking; to cure this, recourse is often had to beer, wine or spirits, which kills the craving for a time. If they ate brown bread they would not suffer much from this and we should be a soberer nation.'

It is tempting to dismiss Graham and Allinson as mere cranks but their views were widely publicised and influenced many contemporary nutritionists.

But battle was not really joined until the discovery of vitamins in the early years of this century. To understand the arguments we must first discuss in detail modern milling and flour refining processes. These are complicated and will be dealt with only in outline.

First, the grain is cleaned by an elaborate array of machines which remove soil, dust, weed seeds and any remaining chaff and so on. One essential process is to use magnetic discs to remove any nails or pieces of iron which may have got into the grain. This is vital not only to protect the milling machinery but also to prevent any spark when metal strikes metal later in the process, for flour dust is highly explosive. Next comes 'washing and whizzing', high speed sluicing in cold water, which both cleans the grain and allows it to take up moisture so as to be in a perfect state for the next stage, conditioning.

We still do not understand all that is going on in conditioning, or 'tempering', but it is known that wheat mills best when its moisture content is at a certain level (which varies with different

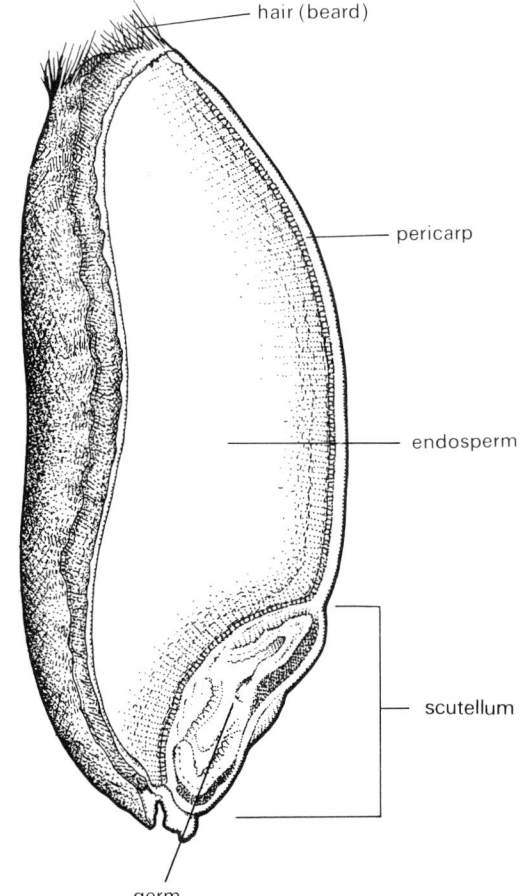

hair (beard)

pericarp

endosperm

scutellum

germ

The parts of a wheat grain.

Composition of 100 grams of flour of different extraction rates

Percentage extraction	Calories	Protein grams	Fat grams	Fibre grams	Calcium mgs	Phytic Acid mgs	Thiamine mgs	Riboflavin mgs	Niacin mgs
100	328	13·6	2·5	2·2	28	242	0·37	0·12	3·5
85	339	13·6	1·7	0·3	19	96	0·29	0·07	2·1
80	341	13·2	1·4	0·1	15	63	0·24	0·06	1·6
70	341	12·8	1·2	trace	13	30	0·08	0·05	1·2

wheats) and if water has penetrated into the grain in a particular way. The conditioner is a container in which both temperature and the flow of air can be controlled. The best criteria for conditioning are reckoned to be holding the wheat for 48 hours at 20 to 25°C with a moisture content of around 15 per cent. If the temperature is raised, conditioning is accelerated and the process can be carried out within a few seconds at temperatures of 70 to 75°C.

Next comes the separation of flour by rolling and sieving. The first rollers, which are fluted and one of which revolves faster than the other, break the grain along the crease and squeeze out most of the endosperm. The outer layers are broken up into flakes which are separated by sieving and passed through another set of rollers to scrape the remaining endosperm away. There may be a third or even a fourth set of rollers and sieves by which the grain is gradually broken down into small granules of endosperm which is known as *semolina*. The separated flakes are bran or coarse wheatfeed.

The semolina is now passed through another series of rollers – smooth this time – which crush the endosperm granules to a fine powder. The oilier and tougher particles of wheat germ are flattened and they are removed using silkcloth sieves, which allow only the flour to pass through.

The final stage of the process is ageing during which the grain is stored for a few weeks. The spaces between the starch grains of the endosperm are filled with a protein called *gluten* and during the ageing period it takes up oxygen from the air, which improves its elastic qualities. Chemicals called improvers are usually added at this stage. These change the constitution of the flour so that it will bake into a large, firm, open-textured loaf.

In general millers and bakers prefer to produce a flour at '70 per cent extraction', that is, it contains *70 per cent of the original grain*. This is the easiest to bake and produces a good white loaf which is easily digestible. On the other hand, some dieticians have argued that 95 per cent extraction, where only the coarser particles of bran are removed, is better.

Such 'wholemeal' bread certainly seems to have nutritional advantages, with higher levels of bone-building calcium and the B vitamins. The table above gives a rough comparison of the nutritive contents of flours of different percentages of extraction. It is only an approximate guide because there will be differences according to the type or blends of wheat used, the soil and climatic conditions when it is grown and the variations in milling processes.

There are variations, too, according to how much of the aleurone layer and the *scutellum* – the 'little shield' layer which separates the germ from the endosperm – are incorporated in the flour. The table below shows the vitamin content of the various parts of the wheat.

Such scientific evidence would seem to indicate that the protagonists of brown bread were right after all and, indeed, they were seized upon with

Vitamin content of wheat grain components

	Proportion of whole grain	Thiamine mg/100g	Riboflavin mg/100g	Niacin mg/100g
Whole wheat	100	0·36	0·16	5·0
Endo-sperm flour	85	0·48	0·07	2·2
Bran and aleurone layer	12	0·45	0·50	25·0
Scutel-lum	1·5	16·55	1·50	6·0
Wheat germ	1	0·90	1·50	6·0

alacrity by those who had previously had to rely on vague notions of health to support their proposition. There is no dispute about the facts: brown bread certainly does contain higher levels of valuable nutrients. But how significant is this?

Let us look, for example, at the vitamin B_1 (thiamine) content. As we have seen (Chapter Two) gross thiamine deficiency can lead to a disease called beri-beri. In Eastern countries, where milled rice forms a major part of the diet and where beri-beri has been endemic, the addition of synthetic thiamine had proved of great value. In countries like Britain, however, beri-beri is never seen, and thiamine is available in many other items of food as well as bread. It is a similar story with the other nutrients present.

Nonetheless, governments have shown concern about the nutritional differences between white and brown flours and taken steps to enhance the vitamin and mineral content of white bread.

During the Second World War, when Britain's food imports were seriously curtailed, the flour extraction rate was increased gradually from 70 to 85 per cent and we enjoyed in our 'national flour' higher proportions of protein, fat, calcium, iron and the B vitamins. Unfortunately is also meant an increase in the *phytic acid* content of the flour. This substance, found mainly in bran and the germ, reacts with calcium and iron to form insoluble compounds which the body is unable to absorb. It was feared that its increased presence in flour could not only make much of the calcium and iron in bread unavailable for digestion but inhibit the body's uptake of those valuable minerals from other food sources as well. So seriously did the Ministry of Food take this possibility, particularly since war-time diets were known to be short of calcium, that in 1943 the addition of calcium to flour was made compulsory. Such 'fortification' is still required by law – and one part of chalk is still added to every 320 parts of flour (strictly 235–290 mgs per 100 grams), although it is now known that much of the phytic acid is in fact broken down by yeast during baking.

After the war reductions in extraction rate were permitted and by 1956 the level had been allowed to drop to the pre-war figure of 70 per cent. In that year a government panel was set up to consider the implications of the consequent re-introduction of lower levels of iron and the B vitamins in our bread. It recommended the addition of thiamine, niacin and iron to flours to bring their levels up to those of the 80 per cent extraction National flour. Such fortification is still required by law: all flour must contain at least 1·65 mgs of iron, 1·6 mgs of niacin and 0·24 mgs of thiamine.

Due to these statutory additions it can now be argued that white bread is nutritionally *superior* to the wholemeal variety. Much of the calcium of the latter is not available to the body since it is present as the non-absorbable *calcium phytate*. The niacin in wholemeal, too, is present in a form which the body cannot use.

Such scientific facts have caused the brown bread lobby to shift their ground somewhat. One form of counter-attack has been to denigrate the additional nutrients because they are synthetic rather than natural. It has already been pointed out that there is absolutely no difference between a naturally-occurring chemical vitamin and one that is produced synthetically but this does not deter, for example, someone like Doris Grant who wrote in *Housewives Beware*: 'It is this very fortification with synthetic nutrients which may present a fresh hazard to the health of white bread consumers and do more harm than good. Although their chemical formulae are the same, synthetic vitamins and minerals have an entirely different action on the body from those occurring naturally as the product of plant or animal.' The latter part of that sentence is totally untrue: synthetic vitamins and minerals *do* have precisely the same action in the body as natural ones.

The problem for the scientist is that he must be scrupulously fair-minded, and he must admit that natural vitamins do not occur, as the synthetic ones do, in isolation but rather in close association with a variety of other chemicals. It is only 60 years or so since the vital necessity for tiny amounts of vitamins was recognised. Might there not be other substances, present in even tinier quantities, which while not being necessary to prevent disease, might help promote positive health? No scientist can be an absolutist and say this is not so. We certainly have not discovered any, even with the most sophisticated analytical techniques. But since it is extraordinarily difficult, if not downright impossible, to prove a negative, we cannot say with absolute certainty they do not exist. To be scrupulously and scientifically fair all we can say is that the possibility is extremely remote.

Those who advocate natural vitamins and 'natural' and 'health' foods are able to exploit this scientific morality. They have a subjective certainty that such foods are nutritionally superior and while they are not able to prove this scientifically, they gain strength from the scientists' inability absolutely to refute their claims.

There is, of course, another way of testing the nutritive values of white and brown breads: their effects on the consumers. At the end of the last war two investigators, Professor R. A. McCance and Dr Elsie Widdowson were given a unique opportunity to do just this.

In the neighbouring German towns of Duisberg and Wuppertal, the population was, like the rest of Germany, hungry, not least because of the scanty German bread ration. The effects could be seen particularly at two orphanages in the towns, where the average weight of the inmates was some nine per cent less than that of American children of the same age groups.

And it was with the 250 children of these homes that McCance and Widdowson were able to make important comparisons of the nutritive values of different types of bread. At the beginning of the study, and for the year of its duration, the children were weighed and measured and given X-ray and blood examinations. They ate normal German rations, largely soups, vegetables and potatoes, but were allowed to eat as much bread as they liked. They had, however, to confine their choice to one of the four different types of bread: loaves made from wholemeal flour, from flour of 85 per cent extraction, from 70 per cent extraction unfortified flour, and from similar flour to which extra vitamins and minerals had been added.

The hungry 5 to 15 year olds ate large quantities of the extra bread they were given and put on weight at a much faster rate than comparable American children, not surprisingly, since they had obviously been undernourished when the trial began. The really significant factor, however, was that the researchers could find not a jot of difference in the growth performance and general health of any of the groups of children, no matter which types of bread they had been eating.

McCance and Widdowson commented on this and similar trials: 'The experiments showed firstly that wheat and flour had a food value for growing children far beyond that usually assigned to it within recent years. The implications of this are great, particularly in parts of the world where fresh foods and milk are scarce and expensive. Secondly, they made it clear that unenriched flour was just as valuable a constituent of the diets used at the orphanages as whole wheat flour.'

Now, just as experiments with Finnish mental patients implicating saturated fats with heart disease (see Chapter Five) cannot necessarily be extrapolated to apply to the general population, nor can trials with undernourished children in the special circumstances of post-war Germany. With the scientist's fair-minded objectivity, McCance and Widdowson were at pains to point out: 'What knowledge had been won? . . Not of course that there were no nutritional differences between the breads, but only that *within a period of a year and under the conditions of this experiment no differences had been demonstrated between their nutritional value.*'

Such experiments, however, are valuable pointers and there is certainly a dearth of information to uphold the contrary view that white bread, particularly that enriched with calcium, iron and B vitamins, is nutritionally defective. One of the fairest summations of bread and the colour problem comes from Allan Cameron in *Food – Facts and Fallacies*: '. . . it is unlikely that differences in the composition of the bread we eat are at all relevant or significant *in the context of our diet as a whole.* Unless new evidence is found it seems that the colour problem for bread is a myth, not of course that this means there are no differences between different types of bread; only that the differences are not significant.'

The Roughage Factor

Our discussion on bread so far has been confined to nutritive factors. Recently, however, a fresh dimension has been added to the brown/white battle, that of texture or roughage. Denis Burkitt was by no means the first to highlight the potential value of bran, or other items of food which give bulk to our diets, but he has certainly become the most important proponent of putting fibre *into* our food.

Dr Burkitt bases his contentions both on epidemiological evidence, comparing disease statistics of populations with high and low fibre contents in their diet, and on measurements of

Condition	In the United States	In Africa
Ischaemic heart disease	Responsible for a third of all deaths	Virtually unknown. Incidence just beginning to increase slowly in large cities
Appendicitis	The most frequent of abdominal emergencies	Virtually unknown in rural areas. Incidence starting to rise in more westernized communities
Diverticular disease	The most common disease of the colon	Almost unknown
Gallstones	Present in some 10% of the adult population	Exceedingly rare
Varicose veins	Present in over 10% of the adult population	Present in probably under 0·1% of those living in a traditional manner. Increasing with adoption of western customs
Deep vein thrombosis and resultant pulmonary embolism	These make hospital life increasingly hazardous	Very rare
Hiatus hernia	Demonstrable in hearly half the population over the age of 50 years	Almost unknown
Haemorrhoids	Demonstrable in nearly half the population over the age of 50 years	Rare or very rare according to degree of westernization
Cancer of the colon and rectum	Second only to lung cancer as a cause of death from neoplasms	Rare
Obesity	Nearly half the adult population is markedly overweight	Rare amongst those living wholly on traditional diets. Becomes common with urbanization and adoption of western foods

rates of digestion and the quality of faeces produced.

His work was drawn together in a paper published in the *Journal of the American Medical Association* in August 1974. He described it as 'the most important paper of my life'. Written jointly with two colleagues, Dr N. S. Painter and Dr A. R. P. Walker, Burkitt's paper concludes: 'Many diseases of Western civilisation have appeared only in the last century. We believe that they owe their origin, at least in part, to the removal of indigestible fibre from the carbohydrate foods that constitute the major part of our diet.

'In the past the physiological function of this fibre has been almost completely ignored, probably because it contributes no calories and has scarcely any nutritional value. This attitude should be questioned as cereal fibre is necessary not only for the "bulk" it provides in the intestine but also for the chemical and biological processes that take place in the intestine.'

Coronary artery disease, say the authors, was considered a rarity in the early decades of this century. Appendicitis, first described in England in 1812, appeared to become common after 1880. There is abundant evidence that diverticular disease of the colon (*diverticula* are small bulges or pockets at weak points in the large intestine) has become a major clinical problem only in the last 50 years. Similarly, Burkitt and his colleagues suggest that varicose veins and deep vein thrombosis really became common at the turn of the century and that the incidence of hiatus hernia, haemorrhoids and tumours of the colon and rectum has increased rapidly in the 20th century. Lastly they say: 'A study of art over the centuries suggests that obesity, now the scourge of Western society, was rare in the common man of Europe until about 200 years ago.'

They make comparisons between the prevalence of these non-infective diseases in America and among African populations, which are summarised in the table above.

The cause of these striking variations, Dr Burkitt contends, is the lack of cereal fibre in Western diets and he says that people who move from high fibre areas to affluent countries are soon at risk from all these diseases, indicating that the underlying cause is due to environmental causes rather than any inherited susceptibility. He shows, too, that the amount of cereal fibre in Britain and American diets has fallen to about one-tenth of the intake in the 1870s.

Burkitt and his colleagues maintain that the physiological reasons for the increased risks of this range of diseases are tied in with the small bulk and longer transit times through the intestine of the faeces. This produces changes in the bacteria within the intestine and gives them a greater opportunity to convert the digestive bile acids into potentially cancer-causing compounds. And the slower movement of the faeces means that such compounds stay in contact with the intestine wall for longer periods. Constipation *is* a fairly common complaint and the JAMA paper comments: 'The modern astronaut makes use of the observation that refining of food leads to fewer and smaller stools, and so he is fed a diet almost free of fibre; this results in extreme constipation with five or six days elapsing between bowel actions.'

There is a further, apparently significant effect: animal experiments have shown that small faeces bulk elevates blood cholesterol levels.

Other workers have come to similar conclusions about the potential dangers of low fibre diets and while much more investigation is obviously needed, there is certainly enough evidence now for people concerned with their health to look closely at their fibre intake.

A switch to wholemeal bread would certainly raise the fibre content of our diets. So, too, would eating more porridge, or breakfast cereals composed mainly of bran. Growing numbers of people are sprinkling a few tablespoonsful of bran on their ordinary breakfast cereals, or eating the stuff with sugar and milk. It is interesting to note here that it does seem to be *cereal* fibre which has the greatest influence on intestinal behaviour. Our intake of fruit and vegetables, which contains cellulose fibre, has actually increased since the 1880s, but their type of fibre seems to have far less effect on the digestive system.

To bake the sort of bread the average housewife apparently wants (or what the bread industry says that she wants) we cannot rely only on the sort of wheat grown in this country. Wheat may be classified according to the chemical structure of the protein in it. 'Hard' wheats are grown in dry climates, and particularly in Canada, while damper climates such as Britain's produce 'softer'

varieties. For a 'strong' white loaf, hard wheats are the best, while home-grown wheats produce doughs which are weaker, less elastic and more suitable for cakes and pastries. Nonetheless perfectly edible wholemeal bread can easily be made from home-grown flours. And perhaps, for economic reasons, we should use more home-grown cereals (see Chapter Seven, page 122).

Where does all this, often conflicting, evidence leave us? Well, literally, you pays your money and you takes your choice. As far as *nutrients* are concerned there is no significant difference between white bread and brown. Wholemeal bread certainly seems to confer advantages as far as roughage is concerned but it will be some time before scientists have worked out all the implications: it may, for example, prove to be better for us to take our bran sprinkled on our food rather than cooked in bread.

Bread still provides some 15 per cent of our daily energy intake and 18 per cent of our protein intake although our bread consumption has been steadily falling in the last few years by about 2 per cent each year. On the other hand wholemeal bread sales, while admittedly being still a very small proportion of the market, are increasing rapidly.

One wonders if, just as the brewers who insisted that the public wanted nothing but gaseous light beers have been persuaded to acknowledge a growing demand for 'real ale', there might not soon be a Campaign for Browner Bread.

But whatever your preference, it is important to remember that bread is an excellent protein/carbohydrate source, both for adults and young children, whatever its colour.

Health foods and food fads

The proponents of 'health foods' have been singing the praises of bran for some years. Now that it appears that there may well be some scientific validity for their assertions, does it mean that other food fads and food cults contain hidden truths?

The answer, again preserving that scrupulous scientific honesty, is that it is extremely unlikely. Some of the regimes suggested by food cults are unlikely to do much harm and might even do some good if, like Yoga diets for example, they lead to a reduction in total food intake. Others, however, could be positively harmful.

But any food cult which claims that the secret of health and happiness is eating one or two 'wonder foods' in large quantities or abstaining from some others because they contain 'poisons' (undetectable in the most sophisticated scientific analyses) should be taken with a largish pinch of salt.

Of all the food cults, vegetarianism is perhaps the oldest and the most widespread. It is certainly true that one can live well enough without eating meat but nutritionists are divided as to whether there are any positive long-term benefits in doing so. We have seen in Chapter Five how animal fats may be associated with heart disease, but many vegetarians go further and claim that meat releases toxic poisons into the blood during digestion. These so-called poisons are presumably *uric acid*, and what are known in naturopathic circles as '*necrones*'. The body itself manufactures half of its uric acid content, irrespective of food intake. The remainder comes from foods such as liver, kidneys, sweetbreads, roe and sardines which are rich in purines, substances which combine with oxygen to form uric acid.

Sufferers from gout or kidney stones, caused by crystallisation of uric acid would obviously be advised to cut down on, or cut out, these foods, but for healthy people uric acid poses no threat and is not known to cause any disease. Those 'necrones' have not been shown to exist except in the minds of naturopaths.

Some extreme vegetarian diets, which may rely more on the aetherial pronouncements of some leader rather than any logical dietary insight, can lead to very serious nutritional problems: scurvy, anaemia, hypocalcaemia, emaciation and loss of kidney function among them. Severe vitamin deficiencies, leading to diseases like beri-beri, rickets and pellagra have also been associated with ill-advised and extreme vegetarianism.

An article in the American Medical Association's magazine *Today's Health* in October 1974 gave these basic guidelines for anyone wishing to adopt a vegetarian diet: 'Cut sugar, fat and oil Calories by half. Replace meat with increased intake of legumes, nuts or textured vegetable protein. Eat more grains and cereals, raw carrots, beetroots, dried fruits and salads. Include cottage cheese, low fat milk and eggs in your diet. To retain vitamins and minerals cook vegetables for the shortest possible time and in as little water as possible. Eat fruit.'

How much meat do you need?

These foods: (av. portion, cooked=3½ oz or 100g)	Give You: (percentage of the protein you need each day)		or, by weight: (grams of protein)
	Man	Woman	
1 Turkey, roasted	50%	61%	31g
2 Pork, loin chop (lean+fat)	44%	53%	29g
3 Porterhouse steak (lean and marbled)	39%	47%	25g
4 Chicken, breast (fried)	35%	42%	23g
5 Lamb, rib chop (lean+fat)	30%	36%	20g

So we do not seem to need as much meat as we are used to eating, particularly if we eat eggs, milk and cheese and vegetable proteins as well (peas, beans, etc.).
Vegetarians lose out on *high quality* protein, so they need to take care to eat a wide range of plant proteins, plus dairy produce and eggs.

Vegans, vegetarians who will use *no* animal produce, including dairy products and eggs, have special problems. For them, says *Today's Health*, it is important to increase the intake of leafy green vegetables and consume a variety of plant foods – grains, fruits, vegetables, nuts – sufficient to meet Calorie needs. Also recommended is the use of fortified soy-milk preparations and textured vegetable proteins and the taking of vitamin B_{12} tablets.

Many health food beliefs have been admirably investigated by John Sladek in his book *The New Apocrypha : A Guide to Strange Sciences and Occult Beliefs*. I recommend this to anyone who would like some instructive further reading. Sladek says: 'Many sects promote some sort of vitamin or mineral supplement, taken as tonic syrup or pills. By thus making the vegetarian a kind of invalid, whose delicate constitution needs pampering with vegetable juices, bone-meal pills, multiple vitamins and herbal tonics, health food establishments cater for the hypochondriacs who probably make up a good part of their clientele.'

But Mr Sladek reserves his deepest scorn for the activities of such purveyors of the secrets of eternal youth and bursting health as Lelord Kordel and Gayelord Hauser, advisers to the Hollywood stars from Greta Garbo to Eva Gabor. Hauser's well-known book *Look Younger, Live Longer* presents his prescriptions for health, which as well as sun baths and massage, eye exercises and sleeping head-downward on slanting ironing boards, include the use of herbal laxatives, enemas and vitamin supplements, all sold by his network of 'Life and Beauty' stores. Hauser lists five wonder foods which, used daily 'can add five youthful years to your life'.

John Sladek says: 'They seem remarkably ordinary on closer inspection.

One: yoghurt, is a delicious form of soured milk containing no nutrients except those in milk. Hauser's ideas on yoghurt seem to be taken from the 19th century Russian scientist Metchnikoff, who thought that the bacteria in yoghurt would replace our normal intestinal bacteria, which, he believed, were poisoning us. They aren't, as everyone but Hauser knew, half a century ago.'

Hauser says that yoghurt comes from Bulgaria where formerly – 'for each million inhabitants, 16 lived 100 years or more, whereas here in the United States only nine in a million reach the century mark.'

Sladek points out: 'I've been unable to find current comparable statistics, but more affluent, degenerate Americans (6·1 per thousand) now live to over 85 than do rural Bulgarians (4·4 per thousand) who still eat plenty of yoghurt.'

Hauser's second 'wonder food' is skim milk, but while this may have uses in a slimming diet and in cooking, it is in fact less nutritious than ordinary milk, lacking vitamins A and D. Foods three and four are wheat germ and brewer's yeast, both good sources of protein, as good as meat or cheese. Mr Sladek's comment: 'They're also more expensive. But then Hauser, who sells them, can hardly be expected to see a disadvantage in that.'

Finally there is black molasses or treacle which Mr Hauser claims is an excellent source not only of B vitamins but also of iron, calcium and other minerals. The *New Apocrypha's* analysis: 'It does contain fair amounts of minerals but not from sugar cane. The chief sources of its iron and copper are factory machinery and boiling kettles; of its calcium, the lime-water used in the refinery. Even at that it contains less of these and other minerals than ordinary beans (several varieties). As for B vitamins, it is one of the poorest sources.'

It has been worked out that the average adult would require a gallon of black treacle a day to keep fit. 'Since treacle is 67 per cent sugar, this would entail a 9350 Calorie daily diet, with a consequent weight gain of around 12 lbs a week (not allowing for diabetes and iron poisoning). Hauser mainly boosts treacle as a source of vitamin B_6, but most normal diets already contain three to ten times the B_6 than most adults need.'

There have been many other 'wonder foods' over the years, from seaweed to sunflower seeds, from royal jelly to silver pills. What most of them have had in common is that once labelled and packaged they seemed to sell at prices far higher than the labour of producing them would suggest is reasonable.

Still most seem to hurt your pocket rather than your health and it is everybody's right to make up their own minds about what they eat.

Rather more disturbing are some of the excesses of a popular cult called Zen Macrobiotics. The cult's 'high priest' George Ohsawa explains that everything in the world is divided into Yin and Yang which 'physically speaking are *Centrifugal* and *Centripetal* force. Centrifugal force is expansive; it produces silence, calmness, cold and darkness. Centripetal force, on the other hand, is constrictive and produces sound action, heat and light in turn.'

Diet is involved because the vegetable kingdom is Yin and the animal Yang, although this division is complicated by salads being Yin and cereals Yang; further clouded by sweet and sour tastes being Yin and bitter and salty, Yang; and totally confused (for me at least) because products from tropical countries are Yin and from temperate and frigid zones, Yang.

Anyway, the idea is always to have a balance between Yin and Yang and surprisingly this seems most often to be achieved by eating a diet composed almost entirely of whole grain cereal (usually brown rice) with the odd salad or meat dish thrown in. Such strict macrobiotic diets have induced scurvy and anaemia, disturbed or destroyed kidney function and led to extreme emaciation in people who were perfectly healthy before they began them.

And the suggestions that macrobiotic diets can cure illnesses or heart disease, polio, syphilis or haemophilia are doubly dangerous: they not only weaken the patient's overall health but dissuade him from seeking prompt medical attention.

Anyone embarking on an out-of-the-way diet would do well to take informed nutritional advice first.

7 Can we feed ourselves

'When we consume a large steak, we are eating something that may have used up enough grain to keep a family in the drought-stricken areas in Africa for a week.'

Kenneth Mellanby, 'Can Britian Feed Itself?'

'Serenely full, the epicure would say, fate cannot harm me, I have dined today.'

Sidney Smith.

'One should eat to live, not live to eat.'

Moliere.

In the earlier chapters of this book we have been much concerned with the current arguments about the *quality* of our food: how, if at all, it should be processed, what may be allowed to be added to it, and so on.

But there are those who believe that these questions are becoming increasingly academic and that our pre-occupation with such nuances diverts our attention from a far more fundamental question. And that is the problem not of quality but of *quantity*: simply, can we produce, and continue to produce, enough food even to satisfy the basic nutritional requirements of the burgeoning world population?

It is a question not only of agriculture but of economics, and recurring recessions increasingly bring the problem nearer home. Escalating food prices mean that a far greater proportion of the average family's income must now be spent on food: there is political concern over the adverse effects on Britain's balance of payments caused by the ever-mounting cost of imported food and altruistic concern over the continuing exploitation of under-developed, primary producer countries.

But how real is the spectre of world starvation? Are we really doing the right things to solve it? And what of our own food problems? Does Britain, for example, need to become self-sufficient in food? In fifty years will the rich variety of foodstuffs we now enjoy have been reduced to a mess of artificially-produced protein pottage and such vegetables as our scarce land resources are able to provide?

The most often quoted, most widely believed, and most disputed statement about the world nutrition problem is that 'two-thirds of mankind are hungry'. It was made, in 1950, by Lord Boyd Orr, first Director-General of United Nations Food and Agricultural Organisation. Almost as soon as the words were off his lips the criticisms began. This statement by Colin Clark, former Director of the Institute for Research in Agricultural Economics at Oxford, is typical: '. . . world hunger is largely a myth, assiduously disseminated for political purposes. The World Food and Agricultural Organisation has staggered from one mis-statement to another.'

He described Lord Boyd-Orr's pronouncement as 'not a deliberate mis-statement but a particularly clumsy arithmetical error' and added: 'Knowing that the statement was untrue, but anxious to preserve the effect, FAO then came out with the statement that half the world was malnourished. On being asked for the evidence on which this was based, they said that it was not yet available – evidently a case of make your statement first and then look for the evidence afterwards. More recently the Director-General of the FAO has stated that half the inhabitants of the developing countries are malnourished. Asked for evidence of this statement, he admitted that he had none to offer.'

I think Colin Clark was being unnecessarily harsh on the FAO and its officials, for the greatest impediment to a rational assessment is an intrinsic lack of fundamental facts: incredibly, *nobody knows what human nutritional requirements really are.*

This is particularly true of the most basic of the nutrients, the proteins. For many years shortage of protein has been seen as *the* major problem and billions of pounds have been spent in efforts to bring protein to the undernourished nations of the world. But has it all been a misguided policy?

The Great Protein Fiasco

'The Great Protein Fiasco' was the headline given to a major article which appeared in *The Lancet* in July 1974. Written by Professor Donald McLaren of the Nutritional Research Laboratory in the School of Medicine at the American University of Beirut, it declared: 'There is mounting recognition that the emphasis which has been given to the role of protein in human undernutrition, resulting in the claim that there is a global protein "gap", "crisis" or "problem", is wrong.'

To understand what has happened we must first delve back into the history of nutritional science. Child malnutrition has been recognised for centuries in Europe and, later, in North America and it usually took the form of what is called *marasmus*. This is extreme emaciation, due to a lack of all types of nutrients, in which the child looks like a draped skeleton. In 1932, however, the first woman medical officer to the Gold Coast, Dr Cecily Williams, described a much different type of malnutrition – a 'deficiency disease in infants' in which 'some amino-acid or protein deficiency cannot be excluded.' It was called *kwashiorkor* which in South Africa means '*the disease of a child when another is born.*'

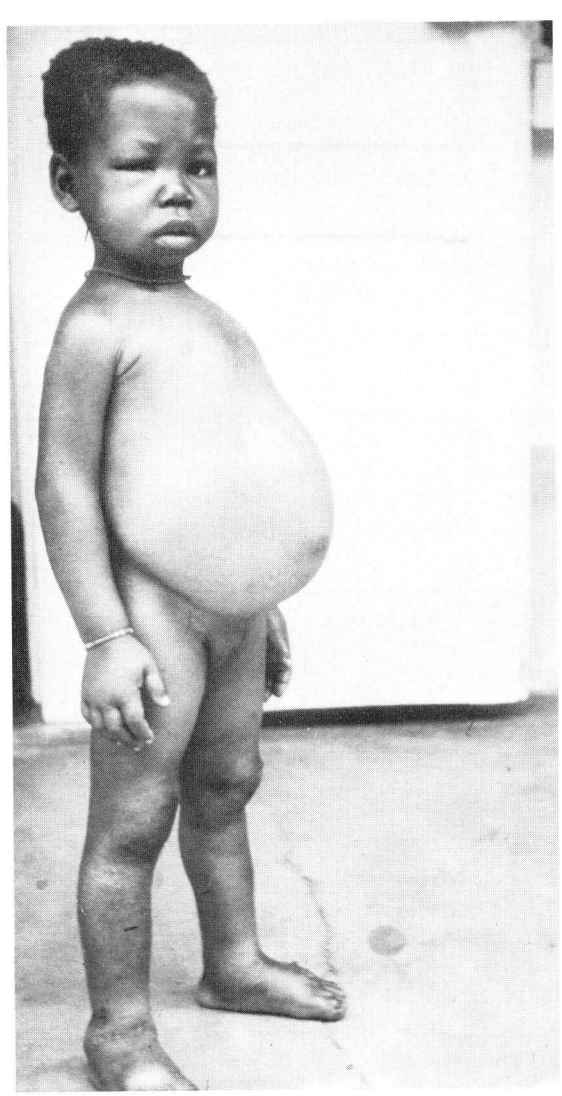

Severe lack of protein can lead to kwashiorkor.

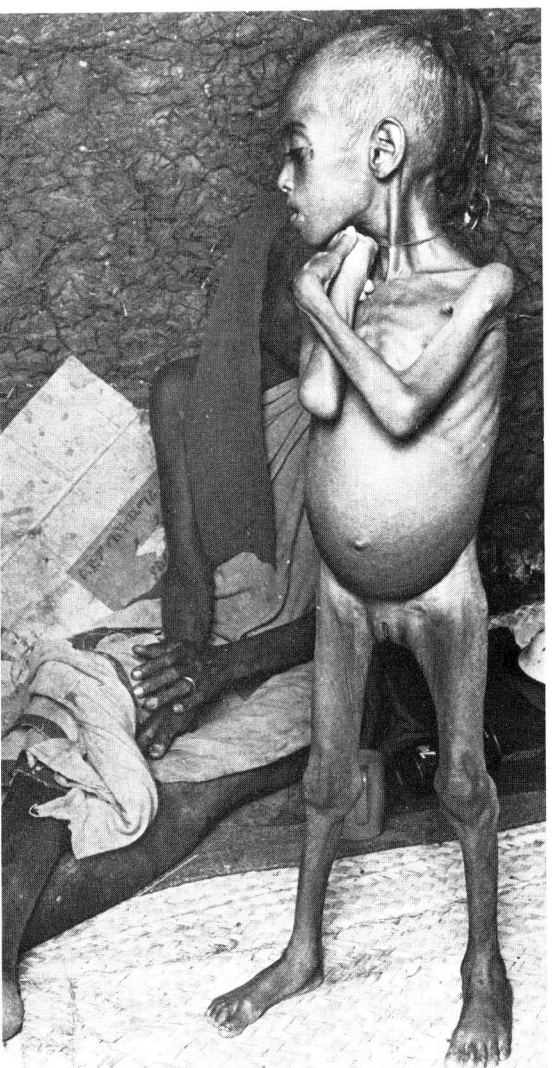

A child starved of all nutrients – marasmus.

It is unlike marasmus in that the affected children do not, at first glance, look thin. This is because their skins and stomachs are distended with retained water. The pot belly is further emphasised by a swollen liver. The victims are particularly susceptible to infectious diseases, like dysentery and bronchitis and kwashiorkor is known as malignant malnutrition because the capacity of the digestive organs is impaired and in severe cases the child is unable to digest any food he is given. Although vitamin deficiencies may be noticeable, the main cause of the problem is lack of good protein.

During the late 1930s and 1940s when there were few international meetings and travel was limited, expert discussion on the nature of undernutrition was carried on in the correspondence columns of journals, mainly between workers in different parts of Africa. After the war the newly-formed World Health Organisation and the Food and Agricultural Organisation began surveys, the most important of which was 'Kwashiorkor in Africa' published in 1952. Professor McLaren takes up the story: 'Without reference to the rest of the world and other forms of malnutrition the authors concluded

H

in a much quoted statement that kwashiorkor "is the most serious and widespread nutritional disorder known to medical and nutritional science". Thus the pattern was firmly set with emphasis on kwashiorkor, soon known as "protein malnutrition", and interest was focused mainly on the rural African scene. Confirmation that kwashiorkor was primarily protein deficiency came with the initiation of cure with skim milk.'

Some workers, however, were by no means satisfied with the oversimplification of the worldwide infant malnutrition problem and emphasised that marasmus, caused by a lack of *all* nutrients, not just protein, was being neglected in the tropics.

Such concerns failed to penetrate the activities of the international agencies whose primary commitment was to closing the so-called protein gap. As Professor McLaren says: 'If childhood malnutrition throughout the world had consisted of kwashiorkor due to protein deficiency, there would have been no fiasco, for the measures taken to identify and combat it would have been appropriate. The whole edifice was built upon erroneous worldwide generalisations made from correct but limited observations in atypical situations such as rural Africa.'

It is now increasingly suspected that marasmus may be much more prevalent than kwashiorkor and since the former condition is due to a deprivation of all nutrients and energy-giving foods, the concentration on protein has been a gross error. Professor McLaren states: 'Dietary factors, especially in marasmus are of second-line order of importance and . . . poverty, ignorance, bad housing, poor hygiene and lack of family planning all conspire.

'Food consumption data and dietary surveys incriminate *energy* rather than *protein* deficit. Increasing the energy intake and not that of protein has produced catch-up growth in children. Lack of nutrients in general with an energy gap rather than a protein gap is the crux of the matter. . .'

Professor McLaren's paper has been quoted in detail because it is of such vital importance to our understanding of the complexities of tackling the world hunger problem. The revelation that protein-deficiency is not the major difficulty by no means implies that malnutrition is a myth but it does show how we can mis-spend hundreds of millions of pounds of international aid in a way

based on a false premise. And while that has been going on children have continued, unnecessarily, to die.

As a result of recent surveys the paper predictions of the size of the so-called 'protein gap' have progressively decreased and the 'saving' is of the order of 10 millions of tons of protein a year, worth at least 100,000 million US dollars. Today, it can be said, the protein gap is not so much closing as disappearing. Dr Philip Payne, of the London School of Hygiene and Tropical Medicine is quoted as saying recently: 'Some nutritionists would say that primary protein deficiency is almost impossible except among people who live exclusively on sago and cassava.'

Until comparatively recently official recommendations for the minimum daily protein intake were around 70 grams, or $2\frac{1}{2}$ ounces. (There are, of course, variations in recommended intakes, to take into account factors like age and sex.) Laboratory experiments, however, show that between a third and a half of this is sufficient not only for protein's major task in the body, that of replacing worn out cells, but for all its other jobs as well.

The implications are far reaching. For example, traditional cereal crops like rice and grain contain protein as well as energy-giving carbohydrates. And if a person gets enough to satisfy his energy needs it seems that he cannot fail to satisfy his protein needs as well. Of course we do know that millions of people simply aren't getting enough Calories for their energy requirements. But it seems that in most cases there is little point in giving them costly extra protein, for an energy-hungry body will simply burn it up, rather than use it for body building and repair.

In other words the multi-million pound worldwide drive to increase protein supplies has been, at best, misconceived and at worst, in Professor McLaren's words, 'a long and disastrous train of events'. It seems that the undernourished would have been better off if our resources had been spent in helping them to increase production and yields of rice, maize, wheat and other traditional crops.

It is salutary to look at the effects that the pronouncements of the 'experts' and the influence of international committees are actually having on starving populations. Three researchers from the London Technical Group studied the nutrition of people in famine areas in Upper Volta and

Ethiopia. In the Ethiopian province of Harerghe, for example, the pastoral population normally has a diet rich in meat, milk and cereals but because of heavy livestock losses in 1974 they were forced to rely much more than usual on wild foods. Their diet became mainly cereals and legumes (peas, beans etc.). Local relief workers regarded it as protein-deficient but analyses by the London team showed that if the local people ate enough to satisfy their basic energy requirements their protein intake would be adequate, even if they had to rely solely on wild foods. Similar results were obtained in Upper Volta.

They reported: 'In view of all this, it is surprising that imports and local production of high-protein foods figure largely in food aid given to Upper Volta and Ethiopia, and in the latter case continue to be recommended by the UN agencies and the Ethiopian Nutrition Institute.'

Much of the high-protein food pledged to Ethiopia was dry skimmed milk 'and some of the remainder were bizarre products, either in context (eg concentrated chocolate whole milk in sachets) or in concept (eg a German product proudly described as 90 per cent animal protein with 10 per cent calcium and probably in fact defatted offal)'.

The London team add: 'Preoccupation with protein is so ingrained among most of the administrators and medical personnel (both expatriate and Ethiopian), and perhaps particularly among those who call themselves nutritionists, that the words *protein* and *nutritive value* have become virtually synonymous.'

The measurement of the true needs of undernourished populations is extremely difficult but a far more reliable assessment could be obtained if resources were set aside specifically for this task. Yet the World Health Organisation, for example, has only just begun to collect worldwide data on all types of energy/protein malnutrition. As Bryan Silcock commented in a *Sunday Times* review of the problem: 'With hundreds of millions of hungry people in the world, a few million pounds spent in finding out how much they really need to eat would be money well spent.'

Human energy needs

Counting Calories, or the measurement of human energy needs has proved by no means an easy task either. In 1973, for example, a group of experts convened by the WHO and FAO 'removed' some 300 million people from the total of those suffering from malnutrition. At the stroke of a pen they revised the official estimate of Calorie requirements for a 'moderately active man' from 3200 to 3000 Calories a day. Official estimates for other groups of people were also cut, and it is more than likely that there will be further reductions in the future, and so fewer people classed as undernourished.

In Britain the recommended levels for that moderately active male are only 2800 Calories, and the Government's own National Food Survey showed that overall the Calorie intake for British families had dropped below recommended levels in the first three months of 1975.

The Survey, published in June 1975, was based on a check of the food consumption in 2000 households. In those three months the average Calorie intake fell to 95 per cent of recommended levels, although protein, mineral and vitamin intakes were still well above the recommended minimums. Much of the decline in Calories was attributed to a decline in sugar consumption following shortages (and *that*, as we have seen in Chapter Five, can surely be no bad thing).

Miss Dorothy Hollingsworth, Director-General of the British Nutrition Foundation, was quoted as saying: 'The figures are clear evidence that food supply is getting tighter. It is a matter for watchful concern.'

But isn't 2800 Calories really too high a figure anyway? Recently surveys suggest that people can function perfectly happily – and work hard – on far less. One was carried out in New Guinea by Dr John Durnin of Glasgow University. He spent two years studying tribesmen and found the average daily Calorie intake for the men, who were much more active than the hypothetical 'moderately active male', to be just 2600. By WHO/FAO standards they 'needed' 3200 to 3300 Calories a day, yet they were perfectly fit on some 20 per cent less.

Even more thought-provoking was a survey in Ethiopia by Mr Derek Miller of the Department of Nutrition at Queen Elizabeth College, London. Peasants there, he found, were able to put in a day's work in the fields while taking in an average 1800 Calories. Admittedly they are smaller in stature than their Western counterparts and so intrinsically require fewer Calories to keep their bodies functioning but such results certainly make

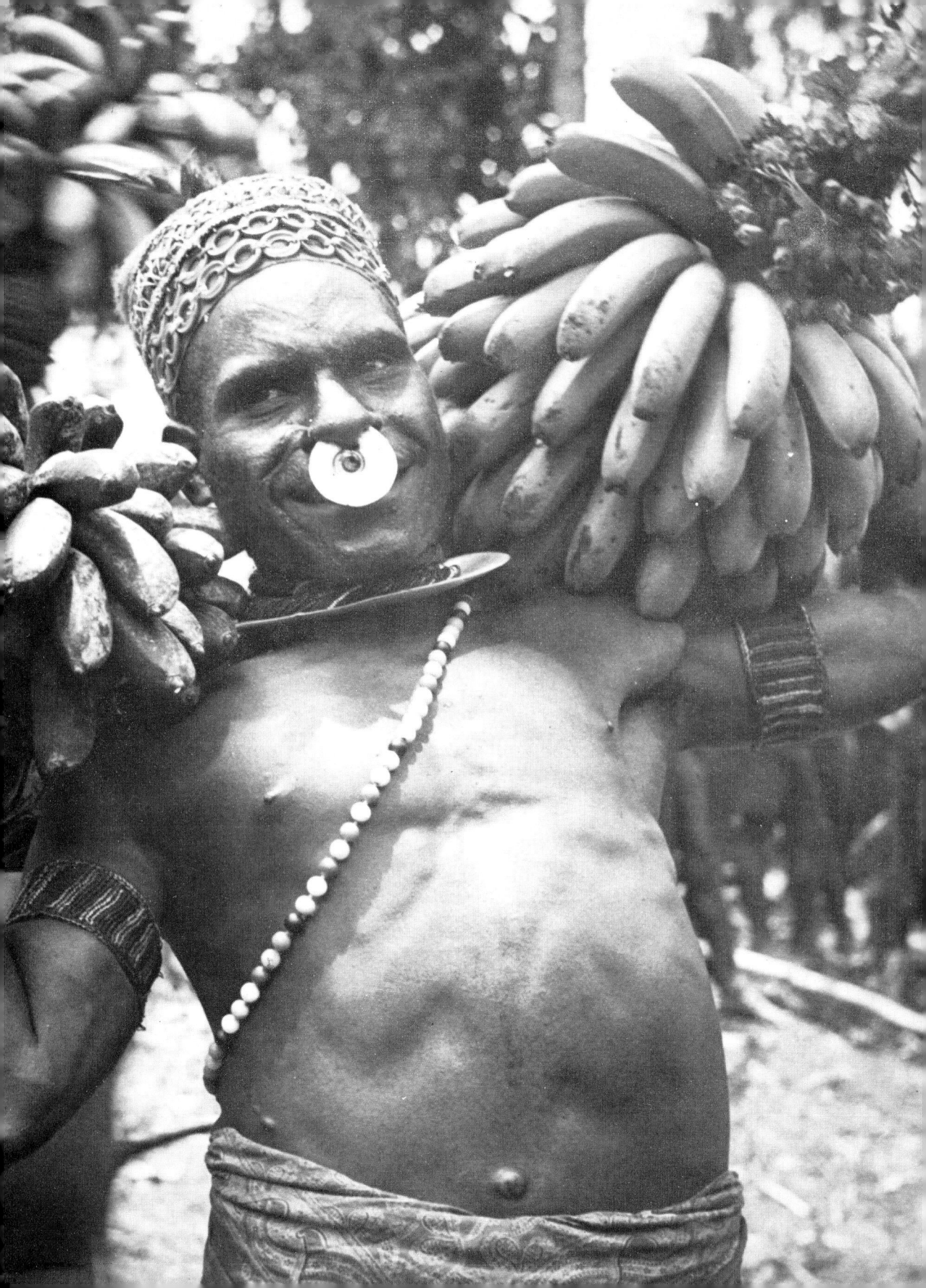

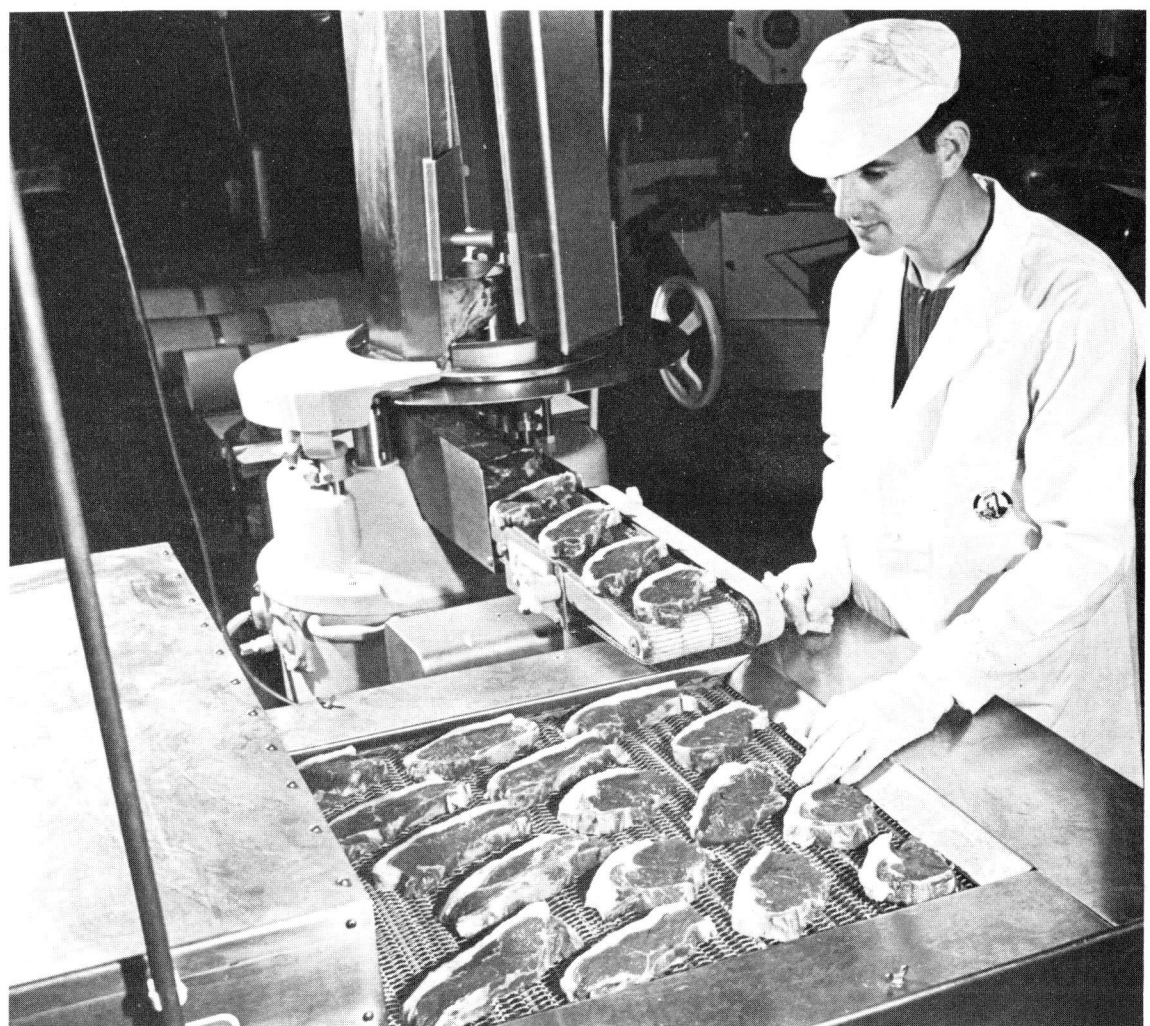

Above. W. European worker: does he need 3000 Calories a day?
Left. New Guinea worker: 2600 Calories a day.

the WHO/FAO official figures seem unduly high.

The facts and figures quoted above are not intended in any way to diminish the magnitude of the task of overcoming world hunger but merely to try to put the problem into its proper perspective and show that solutions are by no means as simple in principle as might have been thought.

It is still true that millions of people are still not getting enough, or enough of the right type of food, to eat. In the past decade for example 100,000 people have starved to death in Ethiopia and another 150,000 in Bangladesh alone. But in

helping them, and particularly in helping them to help themselves, we must be careful to ensure that we are tackling true needs and not hypothetical 'wants', based on inadequate nutritional facts. It is important to realise, too, that Western diet is by no means ideal, in quantity if not in quality. We have already seen the plethora of ills that can be laid at obesity's door and been alerted to the potential dangers of some of the commonest items in the food we eat here, such as sugar, animal fats and dairy products.

Nor should we slip into the easy assumption that provision of adequate food supplies is the panacea for all the problems of existence for the struggling people of 'The Third World'.

Drs James and Margaret Lawless have much experience of medicine, and malnutrition, in Africa. Following Professor McLaren's seminal paper in *The Lancet*, they wrote to the medical journal: 'Much of the drive behind the protein bandwagon stems from the emotional necessity of proving that the miseries of Africa are self-inflicted. The idea that African mothers are not capable of feeding and looking after their children properly is dear to the heart of Europe. Much scientific effort has gone into reinforcing this error. Diet and dirt have always figured in the definition of misfortune, and well-scrubbed virtue is usually cast in the role of provider.'

The Drs Lawless note that many marasmic children remain surprisingly well outside hospital, but in hospital die in large numbers – no less than a third of them in fact.

Kwashiorkor can develop in marasmic children in a matter of hours, usually overnight. Non-marasmic children can similarly develop an acute illness of rapid onset known as *cold injury*: 'An apparently fit or apparently marasmic child at 9 pm can develop into a full-blown case of cold injury or kwashiorkor by 7 am. . . If admitted to hospital large numbers of these children die – 50 per cent of the kwashiorkor cases in one series, 9 out of 13 cold injury cases in another series.'

The cause of cold injury is *hypothermia*, stress on the body systems brought on by cold – and it has nothing to do with protein.

James and Margaret Lawless say: 'This is not to say that there is no malnutrition but it is to warn against the comfortable assumption that low protein explains and accounts for everything. It does not. The killing agent in Africa is the *pneumococcus*. The most lethal environment in Africa is not a village with the customary diet, but a well-scrubbed modern children's ward with an excellent supply of food. The greatest deficiency afflicting the children of that continent is a lack of early access to adequate amounts of penicillin and chloroquine (a synthetic anti-malarial drug).

'These things we can remedy, the alteration of the diet and custom of a whole people is fortunately beyond our powers. Even if it were not there is no guarantee the results would be beneficial. The modern acute general hospital proved a disaster when imported into Africa. It destroyed more children than it saved and provided a bottomless pit for misguided central Government expenditure. Who is to say what the pathological and economic effects of a high protein diet will be?'

If what you have just read serves to illustrate how difficult it is to assess the present situation then consider how much more complex are predictions for the future.

Can the world feed itself?

The first thing we need to know is just how many more mouths there are going to be to feed. Early in the 1970s the predictions were that the world's population would have doubled from some 3700 million (the 1971 figure) to more than 7000 million in the first decade of the 21st century. But now the demographers' extrapolations are looking somewhat shaky. In countries like Britain and the USA birthrates have dropped considerably and in Britain, for instance, there may well be a decline in population. On the other hand birth control campaigns in countries like India seem so far to have had only a very limited success. So 7000 million is merely the best estimate we have got and needs constantly to be updated.

Now it is a 'law of nature' first expounded by the Dutch economist DeVries, that in subsistence agriculture communities both agricultural production and population must grow at the same rate. As Colin Clark, the former Director for the Institute for Research in Agricultural Economics has pointed out: 'If agricultural production grows more slowly than population there will be famine; if agricultural production grows at a substantially greater rate than population, it will be impossible to dispose of it, in the face of the scanty provision in such countries for marketing, transport and storage.'

That this has been true in the developing countries can be seen from the diagram below which charts the growth of food production and population for all developing regions in the two decades of 1950 to 1970. When we examine total world food production and population trends we can see that the rate of production easily outstrips that of the increase in numbers. In sheer numerical terms there are more people now living in developing countries than there were at the turn of the century, despite the fact that many nations, such as Japan, Egypt and some of the Latin American states, have made the transition

118

from a subsistence-agricultural economy to ones based on industry and commercial agriculture. But people living in developing countries now form a much smaller proportion of the total world population.

The considerable rise in agricultural yields has been brought about by a number of technological innovations, including the development of high-yield, disease-resistant strains of wheat, other cereals and rice, the improvement of the soil's fertility with chemical fertilisers, and mechanisation down on the farm. (It is only 45 years ago, for example, that horses, rather than tractors, were the order of the day on most farms, even in countries like Britain.) This agricultural revolution is certainly not an unmixed blessing and poses long-term problems over the conservation of natural resources, particularly of energy.

The current estimates, prepared by the Food and Agricultural Organisation for the UN – sponsored World Food Conference in 1974, are that while the world's population is expected to grow at a rate of some 2·1 per cent per year between 1969/71 and 1985, world food production will increase by 2·7 per cent each year. We have seen previously how disastrously wrong FAO figures and actions can be, but these predictions are based on a far firmer statistical footing than those connected with the great protein gap fiasco.

So, as Magnus Pyke said in an article on 'Hunger and Humanity' in *New Scientist*: 'While famine and hardship have afflicted mankind since the beginning of history and continue to do so in our own times, there is, it seems, no evidence of an impending world food crisis, at least for the decade ahead. From this we can only deduce that where hardship and famine do exist their causes are more justly attributed to the uncontrollable forces of nature or to the vagaries of man.'

'Year by year,' he continues, 'as the FAO calculates, while the world's population has increased, the food supply has increased more. And if this should not be thought sufficient, supplies of nourishing food could be enormously enlarged if, in the richer countries of the world, people were prepared to eat some of the food they feed to their pigs and cattle and (be it said for the wealthiest nations) to their pet dogs and cats.

'It thus seems inescapable that, although science can increase its food supplies, as it has been shown to do, its role is not necessarily predominant in the amelioration of human hunger. . . The cause of hunger is not always technical inadequacy, nor can hunger always be assuaged by scientific and technological means. The solution lies in human behaviour – that is, in the heart of man.'

Man's selfishness – both individually and collectively – means that the Utopia of equal distribution of food resources is still a very long way off. And Dr Pyke's concept of a 'welfare world' where richer countries would continue to over-produce to feed poorer countries pales a little in the cold light of economic day.

For it is a sad fact that the most marked improvements in agricultural productivity so far have occurred in advanced countries: while productivity *has* been raised in most developing countries it has been at a much lower rate. Colin Clark says: 'This state of affairs has prompted some prominent international officials to propose that the advanced countries should continue to produce increasing quantities of food in order to feed the poorer countries. This would mean that the poorer countries would have to produce substantial quantities of manufactures in exchange (unless we assume that the food is to be given away, in which case impossibly large increases in taxation would be required). So far, however, the poor countries have shown little sign of being able to produce such manufactures in adequate quantities – and when they do, the wealthier countries put up tariffs and quota restrictions against such imports.'

The poorer countries, in the meantime, have to pay for their much needed imports and, unless they are lucky enough to be sitting on oil or other valuable minerals, they have to do so by exporting agricultural products in an unfavourable world market – and the subsidised surpluses from the wealthier countries make this market worse.

As Colin Clark says: 'The wealthier countries could help the poorer countries much more by restricting their agricultural production than by continuing to over-produce and to talk vaguely about "world hunger".'

Such a solution is by no means clear cut either: surpluses can prove vital. The Russian grain harvest, for example, failed in 1972 and again in 1975 and only massive purchases from the USA enabled the Soviet Government to feed its people. Over-production may upset long-term economic solutions but it provides often short-term practical ones. (And despite recent record harvests in the

USA there was, in 1974 at least, a world grain shortage so in manipulating the level of surpluses, we have little margin for error.)

Some of the poorer countries, those that have discovered oil beneath their feet, however, have precipitated another crisis by quadrupling the price of their product in a very short space of time. This has rocked the economic foundations of most, if not all, developed countries and caused some radical rethinking not only about long-term energy supplies but also of ways of reducing imports and aiming towards more self-sufficiency.

One question in particular has become much debated of late: *can Britain feed herself*?

Dig for Victory: Part Two?

During the Second World War there was a real danger that the people of Britain would starve. There was strict rationing and every effort was made to increase food production: derelict land was brought back into use, the agricultural work force was greatly increased and in parks, gardens and allotments people responded to the call to 'Dig for Victory'. Despite all these efforts, it is now known, essential supplies ran dangerously low. We still had to rely on imports and had the blockade been a little more efficient we might well have been forced to surrender.

In 1945 the population was 48 million compared with today's 56 million. If we failed to be self-sufficient then, have we any hope of being so now?

One man who believes that we really can – and should – achieve self-sufficiency in food is Dr Kenneth Mellanby, a leading ecologist and former Director of the Monk's Wood Experimental Station in Huntingdonshire. Many other, although by no means all, agricultural experts are in agreement with him.

In May 1975 he set out his ideas in a book called simply enough, *Can Britain Feed Itself?* Mellanby notes that although we are producing more food than ever before we still import almost 50 per cent of our requirements at an annual cost of some £3500 million, 'which is approaching the current figure for our balance of payments deficit.'

Analysing our food consumption Mellanby produces the following table.

At first sight this seems at variance with the statement that we import nearly half our food. We produce most of our own meat, except for bacon, and almost all of our eggs, milk and poultry. Only

Britain's annual food consumption per head of the population in 1973

	Total	Home Produced	Imported
Meat (beef, pork and mutton)	95 lb	71 lb	24 lb
Bacon and ham	22 lb	10 lb	12 lb
Poultry meat	27 lb	26 lb	1 lb
Eggs (number)	245	240	5
Milk	310 pts	310 pts	0
Cheese	13 lb	7 lb	6 lb
Butter	18 lb	4 lb	14 lb
Oil, fat, margarine	38 lb	6 lb	32 lb
Sugar	106 lb	33 lb	73 lb
Wheat flour	142 lb	80 lb	62 lb
Potatoes	215 lb	206 lb	9 lb
Tea and coffee	13 lb	0	13 lb

in fats, both animal and vegetable – and in sugar are there clearly very large deficits.

But Dr Mellanby says: 'What this table does not show is that our meat and poultry, though grown in Britain, is largely fed on feeding stuffs imported from other countries. It also conceals the fact that our wheat and potatoes use imported fertilisers and that all our crops use energy derived from imported oil.'

It is not just oil prices that have escalated. In June 1973 for example cattle feed concentrates cost some £54 per ton; by June 1975, the price was some £79 per ton. And in the same period fertiliser prices nearly doubled, from £24 to £47 a ton.

Mellanby emphasises, as has been pointed out elsewhere in this book, that there is considerable misunderstanding about our actual requirements. When the population eats more meat in one year than was eaten in the previous year, for example, we are told that our diet has 'improved' but 'enough is enough' and if we take in enough for our energy requirements each day it is very difficult not to ingest enough of all the other nutrients. He says: 'It can in fact be shown that we are already producing far more than our minimum basic requirements, even allowing for the special needs of our children and other priority classes. The reason that we need to import so much food is not because we need to eat it. It is because we waste so much to feed livestock to produce meat which, for strictly dietetic reasons, we do not need.'

Nonetheless, we eat not only to ingest nutrients but also for enjoyment and any plan for self-sufficiency must take into account habit and enjoyment as well as basic dietary needs.

One worrying trend has been the continuing decrease in the land available for growing crops or rearing livestock. At least 50,000 acres, and possibly as many as 80,000 acres, are lost every year. About 12 million acres are now left for arable farming. In the last 30 years, however, there has been a remarkable increase in the yield per acre. Between 1885 and the end of the Second World War, for example, wheat production was some three-quarters to one ton per acre; in 1973 the yield was some one and three-quarters of a ton per acre. Similar increases have been achieved with barley and oats.

As far as the cereals are concerned, the acreage has actually increased since the war, from about eight million to nine million acres, largely because of an increase in barley growing. Overall this has meant a doubling of total cereal production since 1945 to a yearly total of some 15 million tons of grain. Sugar beet acreage is more or less the same as during the war but yield has doubled. More than a million tons of refined beet sugar was produced in Britain in 1973. The area on which potatoes are grown has dropped to some 550,000 acres, less than half the 1945 figure and while yield per acre has gone up from seven to 11 tons, total production has dropped from eight to six and a half million tons.

Impressive as these figures may be, many agriculturalists are disappointed with them, for yields on the best farms are often nearly twice the average (three tons per acre for wheat is by no means uncommon) and the average is dragged down by disappointing yields on other farms. Dr Mellanby says: 'It may well be that before the year 2000 we will be able to increase our cereal yields by as much again as we have done since 1945. If this is the case, Britain could become a wheat exporting country.'

Slightly more than half our home-grown wheat is used in bread and biscuit making, the rest is fed to animals. Most of our oats and barley goes for livestock feed, too.

As we have seen (Chapter Six) we need to import 'hard' wheat to produce the type of bread the British housewife and her family appear to like. If we were to eat wholemeal bread instead we could manage without wheat imports.

Turning to livestock Dr Mellanby gives us this picture of the situation in 1973.

The total number in Britain in 1973 was:

Cattle: Dairy cows	3,436,000
Heifers in calf	988,000
Beef cows and bullocks	10,021,000
Total cattle	14,445,000
Sheep and lambs	27,943,000
Pigs	8,979,000
Poultry	144,097,000

Here, too, productivity has increased all round: milk yields have risen from 500 to 867 gallons per cow and eggs from some 150 per laying hen per year to more than 200 today. A broiler fowl reaches in eight weeks a weight that it took a free-range bird three times as long to do 30 years ago. In 1973 the food production count was: beef and veal, 945,000 tons; mutton and lamb, 238,000 tons; pigmeat, 1,018,000 tons; milk, 2,980 million gallons; eggs, 13,368 million and poultry meat, 550,000 tons. But as the Table showed, despite our substantial productivity we are still importing considerable quantities of meat. And although it appears that we are approaching self-sufficiency in everything except butter and bacon, this is a false picture because of the vast amounts of imported grain, and other feedstuffs like soya flour and fishmeal, that the animals are eating.

As Dr Mellanby notes: 'All livestock convert their food very inefficiently. The waste is astronomical.' In the ideal (from the food production point of view) conditions of the broiler house two pounds of food are said to increase the weight of the bird by one pound, one of the best 'conversion ratios'. 'But,' says Dr Mellanby: 'Two pounds of dry high protein food produce a gross increase of one pound in the fowls, but half the weight of the carcase is waste and the other half (or in fact less than half) is meat which is 70 per cent water. So the true conversion ratio is 12 to one, not two to one.'

Cattle and pigs are even more inefficient. Conversion rates are said to be able to reach six to one and four to one respectively: 'The true figures are near 30 and 20 to one when waste and body water are allowed for.'

Only milk and egg production is reasonably

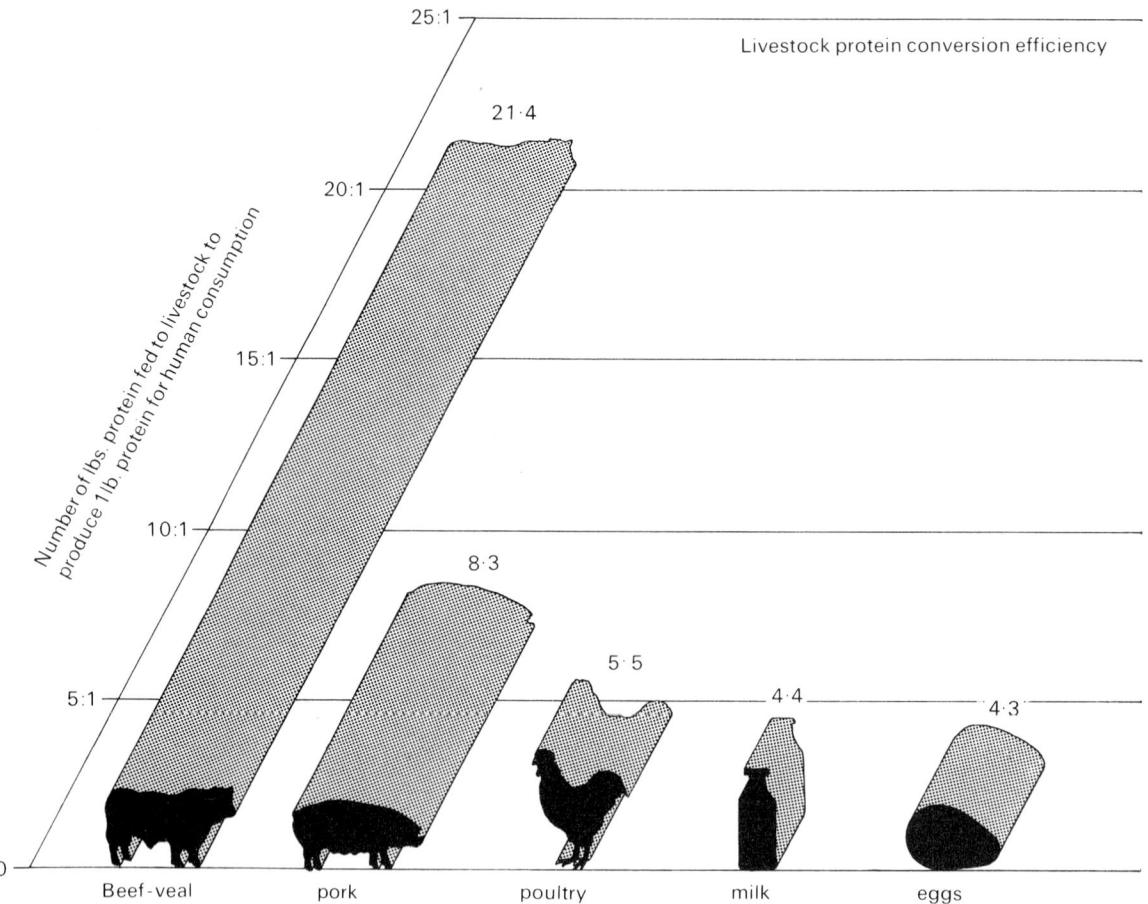

25:1

Livestock protein conversion efficiency

21·4

20:1

Number of lbs. protein fed to livestock to produce 1 lb. protein for human consumption

15:1

10:1

8·3

5·5

5:1

4·4

4·3

0

Beef-veal   pork   poultry   milk   eggs

Foodstuff needed to produce a pound of animal protein. Hens are best, beef worst converters.

efficient in these terms. Dairy cows can give a gallon of milk for every two pounds of food they are given above a maintenance ration, and hens can lay nearly 30 lbs of eggs per year for a *total* food intake of less than 100 lbs.

The main complaint about today's livestock feeding methods is that much of the food would be better eaten by man. 'When we consume a large steak,' says Dr Mellanby, '*we are eating something that may have used up enough grain to keep a family in the drought-stricken areas in Africa for a week.*'

Nonetheless, cattle and sheep are likely to continue as features of our diet simply because they can eat grass which, at present, at least, we cannot.

Summing up, Dr Mellanby says: 'We already produce enough food to ensure adequate basic rations for all. These will be based on the arable

crops which we are growing already. . . . The basic fact in the nutritional picture in Britain today is that we are producing each year some 15 million tons of cereals. If we produced nothing else, these could all be eaten by our population. This would give us two pounds of dry grain which would contain nearly 90 grams of protein and would have a Calorie value of 3000.'

Of course, it would be hard work for the housewife to produce exciting or even palatable meals from cereals alone but it does demonstrate that we can save ourselves easily from starvation with an area of just 9 million acres, leaving another 13 million acres for other crops or good grass plus an even larger area of less-productive grazing land. So self-sufficient Britain would not have to live by cereal alone.

Already potato and sugar production here are adequate to provide everyone with a pound of spuds a day and the wartime ration of half a pound of sugar a week. Our dairy industry provides each of us with nearly a pint of milk a day, and two ounces of cheese and just over an ounce of butter a week.

The livestock situation is complicated. If we maintained or increased the size of our dairy herd, we could expect some four million calves to be born every year, half male and half female. One million of the females would be kept to replace culled cows and a few males would be needed for artificial insemination. So we would have three million calves to rear for meat. Fattening them up on home pasture rather than imported concentrates would take longer – up to three years – and we would probably need some six million acres of land. Taking account of the dairy herd as well, twelve million acres would be needed, or all the rest of our available best land.

But it would produce more than a million tons of beef a year, giving a ration of a pound a week per person, or just over two ounces a day.

If we now juggle our resources, cutting down on grain production, we could give everyone an average 2700 Calories a day in the following way:

Potatoes	1 lb	300 Calories
Sugar	1 oz	100 Calories
Milk	1 pint	300 Calories
Meat	2 oz	150 Calories
Cereal	19 oz	1850 Calories

It should be pointed out here that some people, for example, children, nursing mothers and heavy manual workers may need a higher Calorie intake or more protein. But their needs can be met within the general framework.

The cut in grain production would liberate another four million acres for dietary improvements, and we still have another six million acres of poor permanent grass and 17 million acres of rough grazing.

Sheep, pigs and poultry could be kept (the two latter would not be intensively reared but 'free range' as in the old days). All these calculations, by the way, have not presupposed any increases in yield or spectacular breakthroughs in agricultural technology.

Dr Mellanby concludes: 'The resulting ration would be as nutritious and varied as that provided during the 1939–45 war. It should be remembered that our population was healthier then than ever before or since.'

While it is reassuring to know that, if it ever came to the crunch, we could feed ourselves, it is unlikely that international trade in food and fertilisers will ever cease completely. But given the fact that we are unable to control the prices charged, particularly for imported concentrates and fertilisers, Britain would do well to bolster and encourage her own farmers. As another expert, Dr Kenneth Blaxter, Consultant Director of the Commonwealth Bureau of Nutrition, has written: 'Without accepting the need for complete self-sufficiency, it would be prudent to increase the extent of our dependence on home agriculture through the planning of a support policy. When implemented this would set the base for a further expansion towards self-sufficiency if this ever proved necessary.'

Let them eat grass?

Science, of course, is by no means standing still. Many research projects are under way to improve the yields of existing types of crops or produce more fecund and hardy varieties. But increasing attention is also being focused on ways to exploit the nutrients in plants directly rather than using animals as inefficient protein-converters.

That is why one is apt to read headlines like that in a recent *Times Higher Education Supplement*: 'Let them eat grass'. This was over a report on 'two important and exciting' research projects just started at Reading University. The average yield of protein from beef fed on grass is about 27 kilograms per hectare per year in this country and the theoretical maximum yield from animal protein 350 kilograms per hectare. Obtaining the protein directly from seeds is far more efficient: up to 1000 kilograms a hectare have been produced under experimental conditions. More efficient still is to extract the protein from grass, for in this way as much as 2000 kilograms a hectare – or nearly 75 times the current rate for animal protein – is possible.

Armed with two research grants from the Wolfson Foundation, totalling nearly £250,000, the Reading researchers are searching for the ideal grasses and oilseed plants to provide protein and seeking simple, efficient techniques for the on-farm extraction of leaf protein. It is by no means a new idea: Professor N. W. Pirie at the Agricultural Research Council's establishment at

Rothamsted demonstrated leaf-protein's potential some 30 years ago.

He developed a 'mechanical cow' which transmuted leaves into protein much more efficiently than the natural variety.

The *Times Higher Education Supplement* reported: 'Extraction is fairly simple. Virtually any green crop can be harvested and mashed up, leaving a fibrous residue. The juice contains soluble protein, sugars and amino-acids. It can be fed directly to non-ruminant animals like pigs or it can be fractionated to extract the protein by heat precipitation. One then has three products – the fibrous residue, the precipitated protein and a further liquid residue.'

The protein – it is a greenish powder – can either be used as animal feed or further processed to provide human food. In the long term it is hoped that this latter use will be the major one. The fibrous residue is not wasted, for it can be fed to ruminants like cows (grass may actually provide *too much* protein for their needs). Even the remaining liquid might find a use: it could feed microbes, and yeast could be grown on it.

The UK is at present highly dependent on imports of vegetable oils and proteins. In 1973 the value of imported oil and protein-rich seed exceeded £80 million in addition to imported cakes and meals to the tune of £70 million. Home grown seed crops in 1973 were worth less than £9½ million. As the Reading team says: 'Adequate supplies from overseas have hitherto been cheap and reliable, eliminating incentive towards home-grown supplies, but this situation no longer obtains.'

Several varieties of oilseeds are suitable for adaptation to British weather conditions, among them sunflower, linseed, lupin and charlock, but many problems need to be overcome before they are commercially viable.

The Soya Saga

And what of the humble soya bean? It is an astonishing fact that the USA's greatest single cash export is not, as one might expect, the products of high technology such as computers, but soya. As well as being a nutritionally valuable food, the soya bean is also an extraordinarily economic one: one acre of soya beans, it is estimated, could sustain a man for 2224 days, while wheat would only do so for 877 days, and

beef for only 77 days. The bean itself, of course, is common in Eastern diets, and its extracts are used to make soy sauces.

Already in Britain 3000 tons of soya products are consumed every year, in a wide range of foods from ice cream to pork pies, from cakes to sausages – and consumption is increasing annually. At present, however, still only about 3 per cent of the total soya production is used in human foodstuffs, but even this modest use has caused considerable debate.

There are two modern ways of preparing soya for human consumption: extruding and spinning. The beans are cleaned, cracked and de-hulled and then either cooked and milled to produce a 40 per cent protein full-fat flour or conditioned, flaked and the oil removed, prior to cooking and milling to give a defatted flour, with 50 per cent protein.

For the extrusion process the raw material is this de-fatted flour, mixed with water and colourings and flavourings. The mixture is forced through a shaping die, under heat and pressure, which causes it to froth and expand, giving a textured protein-rich food.

In spinning, the mixture is further processed until it is 90 per cent protein and then forced through tiny holes (about three-thousandths of an inch in diameter) to produce solid fibres.

These are then stretched, to give them elasticity, cut into short lengths and finally combined with starch, albumen or some similar binding substance. This produces a meat-like texture in which the binders break down on chewing but the fibres retain a 'bite'.

The big arguments over soya is whether such products should be used as 'extenders' (that is, they make the meat 'go further') in products such as meat pies, sausages or mince, or whether this textured vegetable protein should only be used, and sold, purporting to be nothing else than what it is. The manufacturers see no reason why they cannot incorporate a product which is at least as nutritious as – if not more so than – the food it is replacing. The Consumers' Associations and the law, insist that meat is meat, and not textured vegetable protein.

It is possible also today to mimic other traditional meaty products, such as bacon and ham slices, wholly in textured soya protein. They are higher in protein and lower in Calories than 'the real thing' – and they contain no cholesterol. But shouldn't we eat soya 'the way nature intended'

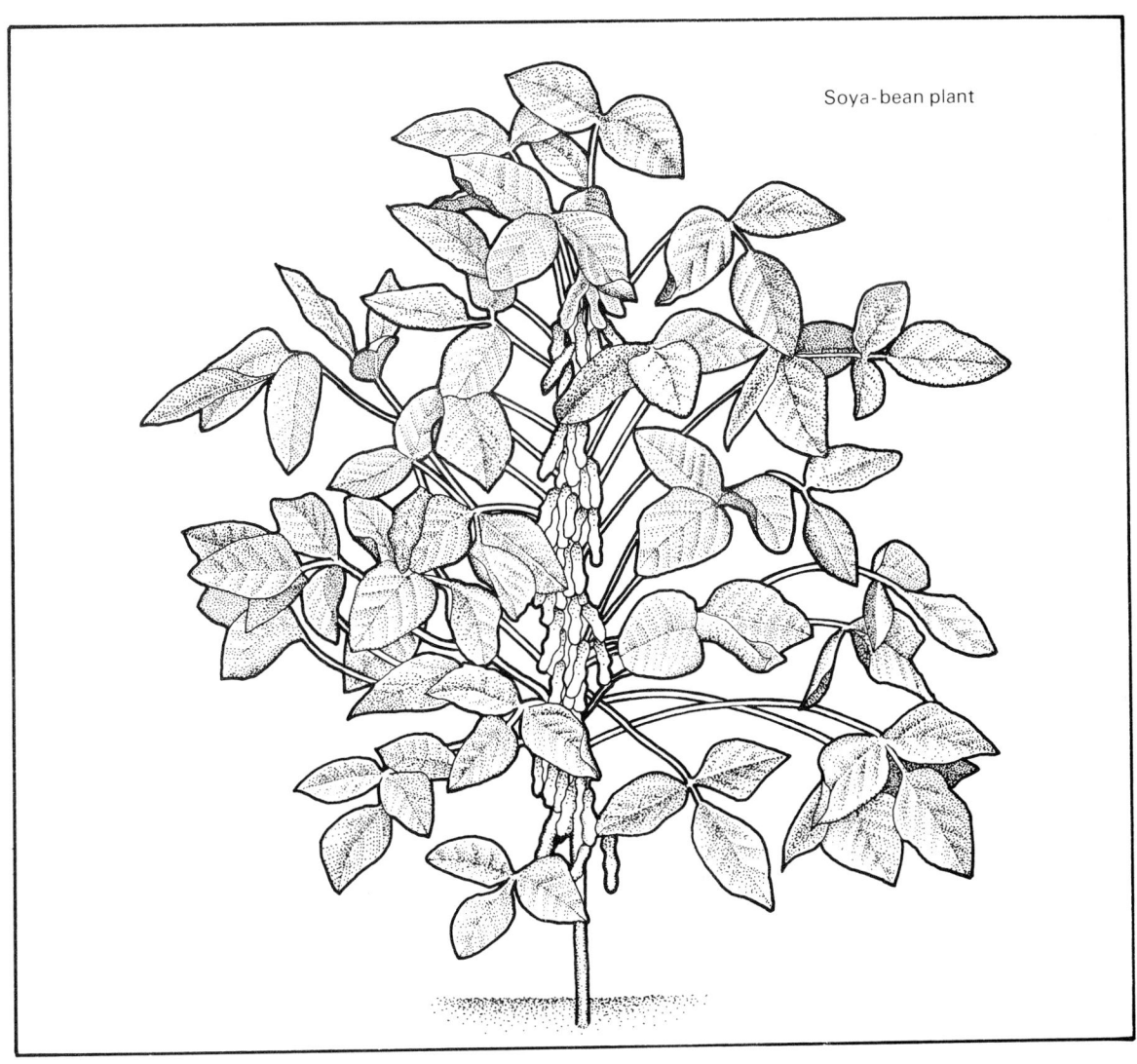

Soya-bean plant

Soyabean: protein of the future?

instead of dressing it up to mimic older, and at present more acceptable, ways of taking in protein? This, too, is the subject for continuing debate.

Nutritionists have called for a more rational, instead of the present rather emotional, approach shown by many people. But the fact is that you cannot change people's eating habits overnight nor can you force them to eat something they do not want.

Textured vegetable protein cannot yet compete with meat as far as flavour, texture and 'chewability' is concerned, however well it is extruded or spun and treated with yeast extract and herbs. And until it does the housewife is still likely to plump for beef, lamb or pork as her family's meal-time protein providers.

Nonetheless soya protein is undoubtedly going to play an increasing role in products where total 'meatiness' is not so important – in hamburgers and sausages, for example – and in meals such as stews, goulashes, mince dishes and the like, where it can successfully be disguised. There is no reason to suppose that the flavour and texture problems will not, in the long run, be overcome. And the escalating cost of industrial catering, in canteens, hospitals and schools, means that it is here that the largest increases in use, particularly as meat extenders, are likely to occur. It will probably be the same story, at first at least, for the leaf proteins developed by Reading University. It is interesting that rules in the USA governing school meals now allow up to 25 per cent of the meat to be substituted by vegetable protein. In Britain, too, its use has become widespread in schools, and vegetable protein has been approved by the Food Standards Committee.

There is no doubt that in the long-term non-animal protein will play a much bigger part in what we eat – and it will not just be from varieties of beans or grasses, either. Throughout the world many research projects are investigating even more unconventional sources of protein, for example growing microbes or yeasts on biological wastes, or using oil or methane gas as the culture medium, and extracting protein from the crop of microbes.

One wonders what Monsieur Brillat-Savarin would have made of it all.

8 Towards more sensible eating

'When we consume a large steak, we are eating something that may have used up enough grain to keep a family in the drought-stricken areas in Africa for a week.'

Kenneth Mellanby, 'Can Britain Feed Itself?'

So far this book has discussed in some detail many of the current attitudes to, and arguments about, the food we eat. We have seen how a thoroughly logical approach to everyday eating is next to impossible because of our ingrained prejudices, our traditions and taboos.

But I think we have also demonstrated that there is a need *now* for all of us to look more closely at our eating habits. In the developed world, for example, there is not only the health hazard engendered by excess and the over-consumption of the wrong types of food, but also the economic problem of providing our needs in the cheapest and most efficient ways.

We need therefore to examine, at international, national and personal levels the food we eat now, the reasons why we eat it and the directions in which we would like to see the inevitable changes in food production and eating habits develop.

This chapter is called 'towards more sensible eating' and in it an attempt will be made to draw together the facts and conclusions of the earlier discussions and give some really practical advice about everyday eating and food purchasing, storage and preparation.

Too often, however, when experts give advice they postulate their own questions and then proceed to answer them entirely to their own satisfaction. But the questions and answers are not necessarily relevant to the needs and concerns of the average layman.

We have tried to overcome that difficulty in the following way: a recent 'Tuesday Call' programme on BBC Radio Four was devoted to the problems of diet and nutrition and several hundred listeners telephoned with their queries and worries. Pressures of time meant that only 15 of the questions could be dealt with on the air but they, and the scores of unanswered ones, do give us a reasonable idea of what people actually want to know, rather than what the experts might think they ought to be informed about.

Of course, there were some repetitions, so we have melded those listeners' queries in some 60 questions, which cover a very wide range of food topics. And our own consultant, Allan Cameron, Head of the Department of Applied Science and Food Technology at the Birmingham College of Food and Domestic Arts, has provided succinct and practical answers. These have been divided into various sections including general dietary concern, vitamins and minerals, proteins,

carbohydrates and cereals, breakfasts and milk, dieting, preparing food at home and processed food.

These were the questions the public wanted answering and this is our informed response.

Section A   General

Is what I, and my family, eat something I should worry about, or if we eat what we like, will we be alright?

The answer really is that if the family eats what it likes and is also healthy, then the diet must be satisfactory and there is certainly nothing to worry about. Perhaps we could just look at what we mean by a satisfactory diet, and to do this in a simple way we can deal with what we call the six main food groups used in meal planning. In group 1 we have got milk, cheese and eggs; in group 2 we've got meat and fish; in group 3 cereals; in group 4 fruit and vegetables; in group 5, fats; and in group 6, sugar and preserves. In order to have a satisfactory diet, then you want some foods from each of those six groups each day using as many *different* foods as possible.

What is a 'balanced' diet?

The answer to this question is very simple and precise: it is a diet that meets all our needs. In other words it's a diet which keeps us healthy, which provides all the nutrients that the body needs in the correct proportions for the body's use.

How do I go about making sure the family are getting a balanced diet – after all, foods don't say on the label how many calories, ounces of protein or whatever, there are in them?

The essence is to have plenty of variety, and as we said in answer to the first question, to include food from all six groups. There is one possible exception and that is group 6, the group containing sugar and preserves. These are really to make the diet more palatable and attractive, but we obviously should not have too much of those foods.

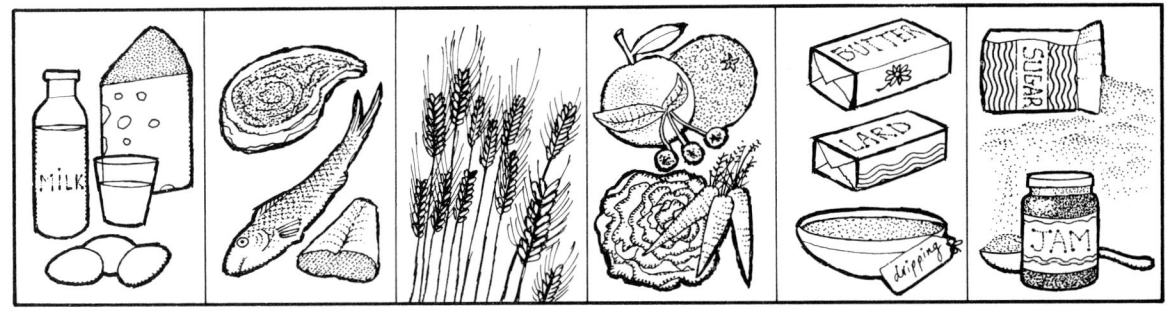

Eat some of each every day · **except these**

If you live alone and have other things you'd rather do, is it necessary to cook much, or even at all, in order to be well nourished and keep healthy?

It is not *necessary* to cook but it is *desirable*. It is enjoyment of food rather than your health which is at risk: without cooking there is a restriction of variety, and to most people a diet without some hot meals would be incomplete and unappetising. But it is worth adding that cooking doesn't have to be a lengthy process and there are plenty of hot meals that you can prepare in, say, quarter of an hour, such as soups, egg dishes, bacon and eggs and cheese on toast.

What are the minimum food requirements to keep, say, old people healthy?

The true answer to that question is that there are no minimum requirements because no one actually knows precisely how much food we need. In the old days, for example, protein allowances were much higher than they are now because we are gradually discovering that people can remain healthy and yet eat less protein than we used to think that they needed. Nonetheless, the Department of Health and Social Security *does* issue recommended allowances of each nutrient, taking into account such factors as age, sex and occupation. This does not, of course, help you in knowing which foods to eat; to do this you have to use food tables. There are plenty of these: the *Manual of Nutrition*, published by the HMSO for instance, contains simple food tables detailing the nutrients in a variety of foods.

Our weekly allowance of essential foods during the war is now sometimes consumed at one meal. Would some mild form of rationing be an advantage to the economy of the nation – and, most important of all, for the health of the people?

The first thing to make clear is that there simply is no such thing as an essential food. There is no such thing as a perfect food either, although some foods, such as milk, come fairly near that ideal. The effect of rationing was to cut down consumption of certain foods, rather than cause us to eat *essential* foods. It forced us to cut down on sugar, sweets and sugar-containing foods whereas today we tend to eat too many of such foods. War-time rationing also cut down on fats and it was these that people missed most, for they help to make a meal really palatable. Today there is fairly strong evidence to suggest that we should be careful about eating fats, particularly animal fats, and that many of us really ought to cut down on

We were thoroughly healthy on wartime rations.

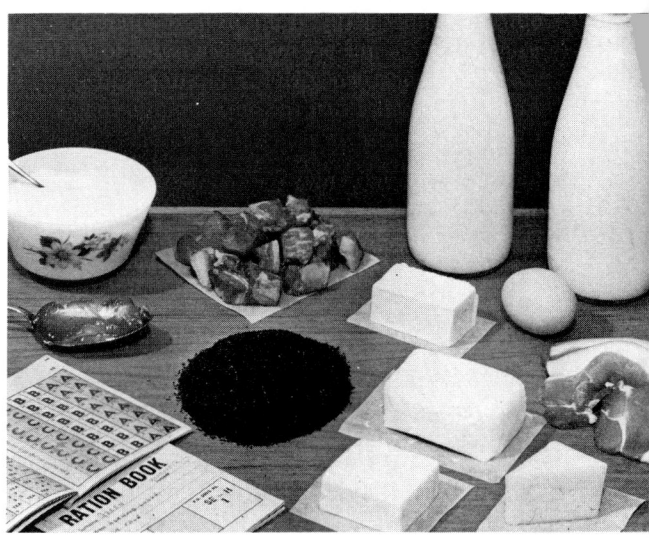

J

fat consumption. Our problem now is eating *too much*, so the real answer to the question is yes; rationing could force us to cut consumption of foods we would be better off without. But whether anyone would accept it in peace time is very much in doubt.

Are there too many useless foods, such as biscuits and cornflakes, on the market?

This is a loaded question because the examples quoted, biscuits and cornflakes, certainly aren't useless. They are however, typical convenience foods and they do encourage too high a consumption of sugar. Our increasing dependence on such convenience foods may cause us to have too much carbohydrate in our diet, which is the nutrient that most of us could do with less of.

I'm concerned that the nutritional value of food is being spoiled by germ contamination during preparation. The TV cooks are encouraging this bad habit, which is serious, since tummy upsets are the second highest cause of absence from work and this could be prevented by better kitchen hygiene. What can be done about this?

First of all, we need to make the point that there is a confusion within the question, because germ contamination during preparation has got nothing to do with nutritional value of the food. You can have contaminated food which still has a high nutritional value. That does not mean that food hygiene isn't most important in the home, but I can't agree that we can blame TV cooks for bad hygiene. Good hygiene will certainly prevent contamination of food during preparation, and improved standards can only come through teaching of the principles of hygiene and by – and this is most important – practical example in places where the food is being prepared, such as schools, homes and even, of course, on the TV screen.

The rules of hygiene are really common sense. Once you understand that all foods deteriorate once they have been harvested or prepared and that there are germs in the kitchen on every surface and in the air, then you can begin to appreciate that cleanliness in *every* aspect of food preparation is the basis of good hygiene.

Healthwise, is it true that 'a little bit of what you fancy does you good'?

It is partly true and partly false. Many people who eat what they like do have a varied and balanced diet that keeps them perfectly healthy. So for such people, a little bit of what they fancy certainly does them good. But there are also many people whose diet doesn't keep them as healthy as they should be. Obesity is an obvious example. Here people are often over-eating an unwise selection of food and for them the old adage certainly is not true. If you are going to have a little of what you fancy the emphasis should be on *a little*.

Is irregular diet a bad thing? Does one have to eat three times a day?

This is rather difficult to answer. In this country most people have three regular meals a day and this is a satisfactory way of life. But there is certainly no law about it, because the body does adapt to other regimes quite quickly, so you could have a perfectly satisfactory diet eating two times a day or four times a day. Of course in other countries people do have completely different dietary regimes. However *often* you eat, though, *regularity* in meals is helpful to the smooth running of body mechanisms.

Is a snack as good as a hot meal?

	Weight (oz)	Protein	Fat	Calories
Snack				
Roll	3·5	5·4	1·4	252
Butter	0·3	0·3	7·0	63
Cheese	2·0	14·2	19·6	234
Tea	10·0	1·0	1·0	50
Orange	2·0	0·4	0	20
Hot meal				
Mutton	2·4	9·0	21·0	225
Cabbage	3·0	1·2	0	21
Potato	4·0	2·4	0	84
Apples	3·0	0·3	0	36
Custard	2·0	1·8	2·2	66
Totals				
Snack		24·3	29·0	619
Hot meal		14·7	23·2	402

Should children have a cooked meal every day?

If we give a nutritional answer to that question, then the answer is no, but on the other hand, in order to have a varied and attractive diet, the answer is probably yes. But again there is no law about it, and it's important for mothers to appreciate that sandwiches, picnics, these sort of meals, can have just as much food value as a cooked meal of meat and two veg. Many people may feel sandwiches are fattening compared with the latter type of meal but this can be completely untrue. If you have a hot fried meal, for example, this can contain far more Calories than, shall we say, sandwiches containing beef, tomatoes and lettuce.

Section B   Vitamins and minerals

Do you think that if one has an adequate and sensible diet it is necessary to buy vitamins, pills, etc. that are so widely advertised and so very expensive. Who, if anyone, needs extra vitamins?

The answer to the first part of that question is, as emphatically as I can put it, no. If you do have a sensible diet there is absolutely no need to buy vitamins and pills, in fact there is every reason *not* to do so. More and more these days we are learning that over-consumption of vitamins can have undesirable consequences *(see next question).*

The answer to the second part of the question is that hardly anyone in this country needs extra vitamins. There are one or two possible exceptions, mainly among the very young and the very old. For example, babies fed on cows' milk, or preparations based on cows' milk, may be short of some vitamins, but again, there is no reason for them to be given vitamins or pills. They can get their extra vitamin C from orange juice and their vitamins A and D from cod liver oil.

I think there is a great deal of misunderstanding about vitamins in food. Certain foods contain one vitamin, other foods contain a different one, and what we need is regular small quantities of *all* the vitamins, so we are back again to the maxim of eating as varied a diet as possible.

What quantities of vitamins does one actually need in a diet? For instance, is one glass of orange juice enough per day, or should one drink two? How can we be sure we don't end up spending more (or less) than we need, and are there dangers in too many vitamins?

First of all, you may hear some people talking about foods that are full of vitamins, but this is a complete fallacy. The actual amounts of vitamins in any food are very small indeed. This is not important because the quantities we need in the diet are also extremely small. Let's take the

example of a glass of orange juice. The juice is a good source of vitamin C and one glass will provide us with all the vitamin C that we need for a day. But that does not mean that one *has* to drink a glass of orange juice a day. The main source of vitamin C in our diet is potatoes, and if we included them in just one meal we would probably take in enough for our daily needs.

Regarding the dangers of over-consumption, there are very real dangers of certain vitamins being taken in too large amounts, particularly those vitamins which are soluble in fat and which can be retained by the body, namely vitamins A and D. Recently there has been an interesting example of this, where a man actually died of over-consumption of vitamin A which he obtained by drinking extremely large quantities of carrot juice. Not content with that, he supplemented his diet with vitamin A tablets, and the result was disastrous. We can, however, reassure people that it would be very difficult for somebody eating sensibly to get too many vitamins. It is only vitamins A and D that can cause problems, and one would really have to be as silly as that man was to take in enough to do harm. In the ordinary diet there is no danger of over-consumption of vitamins.

Where to get Vitamin C

Food Source	mg per oz
Rose-hips	700
Black-currants	57
Green Peppers (raw)	36
Brussels Sprouts (raw)	28
Brussels Sprouts (boiled)	10
Cabbage (raw)	17
Cabbage (boiled)	6
Potatoes (raw)	2–9
Potatoes (boiled)	1–4
Potatoes (chips)	2–6
Potatoes (roast)	2–7
Tomatoes	6
Lettuce	4
Apples	1

Is there any truth in the theory that one can be protected against heart attacks by taking vitamin C tablets daily?

To my knowledge, there's no truth in this, but perhaps we need to make the point that there certainly is an established relationship between heart disease and diet, though to date the exact nature of this link is not proved. So any claims at present that we are protected against heart attacks by taking any one nutrient or any one sort of food is really no more than a theory. There is absolutely no conclusive evidence.

Do large doses of vitamin C help you stop getting colds?

Again there is absolutely no conclusive evidence that large doses of vitamin C stop you getting a cold nor that once you have got a cold, large doses of vitamin C will help cure it. But an eminent scientist in America, Dr Pauling, who is a double Nobel prize winner, has claimed that large doses of vitamin C cure his colds, and many other people have taken up his idea. Having said that the old adage that 'a cold lasts seven days if you treat it, and a week if you leave it alone' still seems to be true. Extra vitamin C certainly will not do you any harm.

I used to know someone who would drink the vegetable water after cooking, as he said it contained all the vitamins that had been boiled out. Is it true that this water has all the vitamins in it?

First of all, when we are talking about *vegetables*, we need to realise that the only vitamin that we are really concerned with is vitamin C. So I wouldn't say water has *all* the vitamins in it; the only possibility is that it might have vitamin C in it. But the suggestion is partly true because vitamin C is soluble in water, so when vegetables are cooked there will be some loss of the vitamin into the cooking water. It is, therefore, good practice to use the cooking water. I would not suggest drinking it which would be extremely unpleasant, but using it for making gravy or as a basis for soup or stews.

To preserve the vitamins in fruit juice, should one squeeze oranges at the very last moment? Has the vitamin C been destroyed in a carton that has been sitting on a shelf for some time? Is tinned fruit juice as good a source of vitamin C as fresh?

The thinking behind this question is correct, namely that fruit juice is a valuable source of vitamin C and that vitamin C, above all other vitamins, is the one that tends to get destroyed. It is destroyed in various ways, but one way is certainly on storage in air. So although I think it would be unrealistic to squeeze an orange at the

very last moment before you drink it, it is true that if you left it for a long time, then it would lose some of its vitamin C.

To give another example, milk does not contain much vitamin C, but milk which is left on a doorstep in the sunlight for several hours will certainly suffer a *reduction* of its vitamin C content.

Vitamin C is also lost when foods are heated and when they are in contact with the air, so that by keeping food at low temperatures, such as in the refrigerator, and by keeping it in sealed containers, we can help to reduce the loss of vitamin C.

The last part of the question asks whether tinned orange juice (and I suppose frozen orange juice as well), is as good as the fresh product. In terms of quality, it may not be so 'good' in the sense that it will taste different and it may well contain a preservative or other additives, but in terms of the vitamin C, it is likely that the tinned or the frozen juices will contain just as much as the so-called 'fresh' orange, especially if you consider how long it has been since that orange was on the tree. Sometimes, too, the tinned and frozen juices will have extra vitamin C added, which means you may be getting *more* than in the fresh juice.

How far are vitamins destroyed by canning, particularly in fruit?

Here again we are dealing largely with vitamin C because this is the vitamin present in fruit and most vegetables. The straight answer is: Yes, we do lose vitamin C during canning, because during the process the food is heated, and even more vitamin C is lost by oxidation which occurs in the can on storage. Despite this, however, the canned fruit or vegetable may still contain more vitamin C than the so-called 'fresh' equivalent, because the fresh equivalent can take a long time to get to the shops and to your kitchen.

What is the importance of vitamin B? Are there more B vitamins than those added to cornflakes?

There are a whole range of B vitamins, seven in all, and their importance in the body is that they are concerned with energy release. There certainly are more B vitamins than those you find in cornflakes. Perhaps we should add too that eating cornflakes is not an economical way to get vitamin

Where to find Vitamin B

	Thiamine	Nicotinic Acid	Riboflavine
Good sources	Dried Yeast Wheat germ Peanuts Lean pork Kidney Wholemeal flour	Dried yeast (and extract) Liver Kidney Meat extract Wheat germ Cocoa Cheese Eggs	Meat extract Yeast extract Liver and kidney Meat Wheat germ Wholemeal flour Chocolate
Moderately good sources	Meat Walnuts Chestnuts Fish Eggs Potatoes Greens	Spinach Dried apricots Milk Oatmeal Fish Brown bread Beer	Peas and beans White flour Polished rice Oatmeal Dried fruit Chocolate
Poor sources	White flour White rice Jam Sugar	Maize Meal Polished rice White bread Fruit Jam Sugar	Maize Meal Potatoes Green vegetables Fruit Milk Eggs Cheese

B or other vitamins. It is better to eat foods like milk, cheese, eggs, meat and fish which are good sources of B vitamins.

How important is the mineral content of foods?

It is very important in the sense that minerals are essential to the healthy working of the body. But there is generally no need to worry about mineral intake because any varied diet provides us with adequate supplies since minerals are distributed through a very wide range of foods. The only people who may possibly go short are those in very special circumstances. People who live far away from the sea, particularly if they don't manage to obtain any sea food, might just possibly be short of iodine, for example. To cover this eventuality some salt has iodine added to it. Such iodised salt can readily be bought in shops.

Children, of course, need larger than normal supplies of some minerals, particularly calcium, when they are growing. This is why there's such an emphasis on milk in diets for young people, because this does supply a good balanced supply of vitamins and minerals. For growing children a pint a day is ideal.

Section C   Proteins

We are told that meat is an expensive way of getting protein. In what other ways, for example cereals, should we be able to get protein? And is this sufficient?

Well, it's true that meat is an excellent (though expensive) protein source. It is also true that cereals are an alternative way of getting the protein that we need. In this respect we might single out bread, which is not normally thought of as a protein food but which, in fact, supplies us with a considerable proportion of the protein in our diet.

Thinking of foods other than meat which are good suppliers of protein, then apart from bread, which is the best buy in terms of nutrients for money spent, the next best would be cheese, followed by milk and then eggs.

Value for money in protein

16p buys (Nov. 1975)	Protein (g)	Calories
28 oz white bread (sliced/wrapped)	61·6	1,932
5·8 oz Cheddar cheese	41·8	696
5½ standard eggs	37·4	506
1·9 pints milk	29·8	628
4·7 oz stewing beef	25·9	235
4·4 oz fresh cod	22·4	101
2 lb 5 oz old potatoes	14·7	847
8·3 oz butter	0·8	1,876

Our family, both parents and children, is not very keen on meat. Am I, as a mother, doing the right thing to encourage or even force them to eat these foods?

From a nutritional point of view, and also from a cost point of view, the answer is certainly no. There are plenty of other foods that can replace meat in the diet – cheese and eggs for instance – and you can save a good deal of money by giving alternative foods.

Now that we are being introduced to soya bean products, is there a possibility that we could have protein in excess of our needs?

It is true that soya bean protein products are a useful source of protein and very often they are used as what we call *protein extenders*, that is, they are used in conjunction with meat in such things as stews and curries. It is also true that most of us do take in quite enough protein for body-building needs, so there's no need to have additional protein from soya bean products. On the other hand, there's no *danger* of having too much protein because any excess in our diet is simply burned up for energy, or converted to fat.

Can you give advice about balancing complementary proteins to get all the necessary amino-acids?

There are certain amino-acids, the chemical 'building blocks' of all proteins, which we call *essential*: that is, our diet must supply us with them because the body cannot actually make them for itself. So in choosing a diet, we want to make sure that we receive enough of all these essential amino-acids, of which there are eight. The simple rule for doing this is to eat animal protein *along with* vegetable protein. These two complement each other and give us all the essential amino-acids. In other words, tried and tested favourites such as fish and chips, egg and beans, macaroni cheese, and similar dishes are all good choices from this point of view. Of course, when I say *animal* protein, I am not specifically referring to meat, I am also including all animal sources, dairy sources, fish, and so on.

How much protein do we need, in our daily diet? How much meat, bacon or sausages, for example, should we eat at one meal?

As we said previously no one actually knows what our protein needs are. What *is* certain is that, in this country, most of us are getting at least as much as we need to keep us healthy. Coming to the question of how much protein at one meal, the general principle here is 'a little and often'. The body does not store protein. Therefore, if we have small amounts of protein in each meal, it enables us to make the best use of it for body-building and not 'waste' it in producing energy or in turning it to fat.

Where do we get our protein?

The sources of protein in the British diet	%
Bread, flour etc.	40
Dairy Produce	20
Meat	17
Fish, poultry	6
Potatoes	6
Eggs	4
Vegetables and other foods	7
	100

Very roughly, the amount of protein required for a woman is two ounces a day, and for a man is three ounces a day. Of course meat, for example, is not solid protein: a quarter ounce (100 gramme) portion of meat would provide a woman with about a quarter of her day's protein. The other three-quarters of her protein requirements should come from other sources including cereals and vegetables.

Will a vegetarian diet give us all the protein, and other nutrients, that we need?

Vegetarians certainly seem to exist very happily on the diets they choose and most live healthy lives. On the other hand, if vegetarians are strict and exclude milk, cheese and eggs from their food, there is a real problem in planning a diet which provides enough protein because such a diet, relying heavily on vegetables and nuts, is likely to be very bulky and rather monotonous. It can be done, but in my view it is not a desirable thing to try to do because the diet is never going to be very varied and never going to be very attractive.

Section D   Carbohydrates and cereals

So much is heard about the ill-effects of too much sugar. Is this true?

An emphatic yes. In general too much of any one item of the diet is unwise and our consumption of sugar has increased about five-fold over the last hundred years, so that today in an average lifetime we consume some 50 cwt of sugar, an astonishing and somewhat alarming thought. Over-indulgence in sugar is certainly bad for our health for a number of reasons: it's bad for our teeth, it's bad for our figures and it may well have

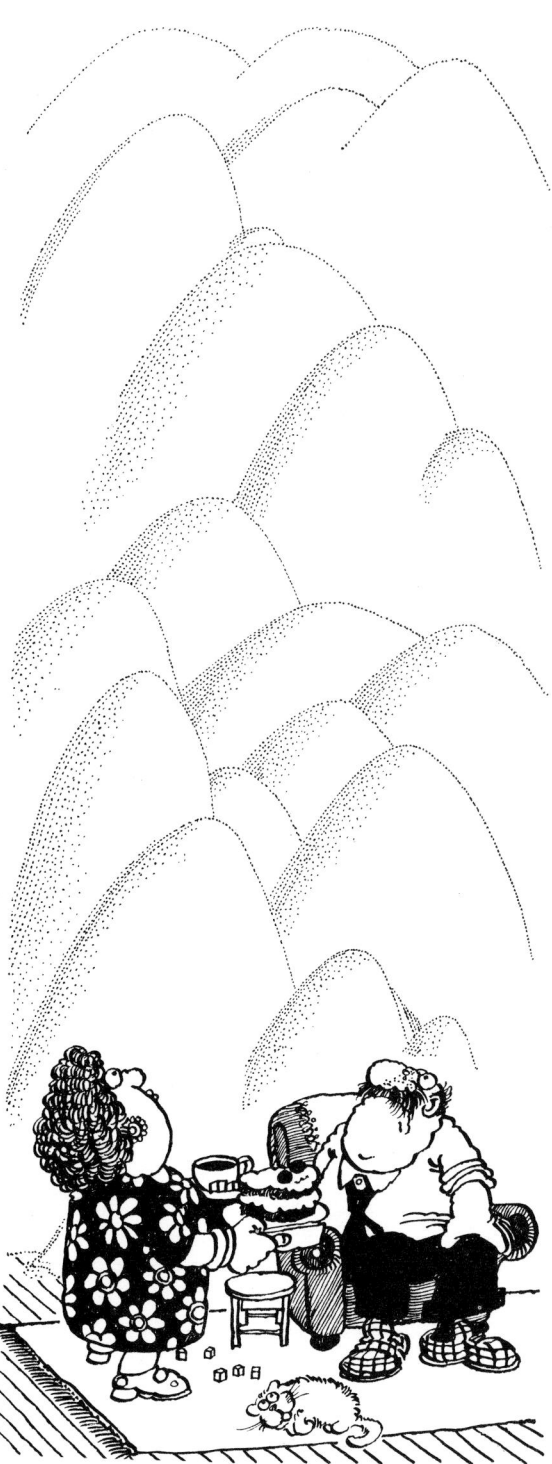

A man eats 50 cwt of sugar in a lifetime.

a connection with heart disease. Many of us do have a sweet tooth, but to a large extent this is because of bad habits we have formed in infancy and it's a matter of strong will to overcome these bad habits. You have just got to stick it out and reduce your intake by not putting sugar in tea and coffee and other beverages, by not adding so much sugar to fruit and other foods. If you cannot stand them without sugar, then there is no reason at all why you shouldn't replace the sugar with saccharin. I know it has the disadvantage of a slight bitter after-taste but it is certainly, from a nutritional point of view, a wise thing to do.

You can also buy low-calorie foods; I'm thinking, for example, of products such as fruit squashes, where a large proportion of the sugar which is normally present is replaced by saccharin.

It is debatable whether it is better to stop using sugar in beverages at a stroke or to try to cut down gradually. I think this has to be a personal choice. I personally would prefer the short, sharp method. In fact this is something I have done and now I can't stand sugar in tea or coffee.

I think the sugar problem is so important that if the readers of this book decide to make one resolution about their diet, then it should be that they will reduce their sugar intake. Nothing else is so sure to have a beneficial effect.

I have heard that brown sugar is better than white. Is that true? And is honey better than either?

No, that is a complete fallacy. White sugar is simply refined to a greater extent than brown, but basically they are both the same substance, that is, sucrose. There is nothing magical in brown sugar nor anything particularly desirable. Honey simply contains *two* basic sugars, glucose and fructose. When we digest ordinary sugar (sucrose) we break it down to glucose and fructose. So, as far as the body systems are concerned, they are getting the same substance. Of course, you may prefer honey for quite a different reason and that is because it is more palatable and more attractive.

To what extent is white bread and white flour a health hazard?

I think it would be fair to say that it is not a health hazard at all. In fact, the first point I would like to make is that considering value for money, white bread is the most useful food on the market today, and it's also one of the most underestimated foods in our diet.

The implication in the question is that it is white bread as *opposed* to wholemeal bread that is a health hazard, and this again is a nonsense. What *is* true is that modern diets tend to lack roughage or fibre, and in this particular respect, white bread is inferior to wholemeal bread. Wholemeal bread contains about two per cent of fibre or roughage. Brown bread must, by law, contain at least 0·6 per cent, whereas white bread contains only a trace. It is however, illogical to blame the lack of fibre in our diet on white flour, on white bread. As time has gone by and we have become more dependent on convenience foods which are processed in one way or another, we tend to have lost fibre from natural foods. For example, wheat grains and other cereal grains do contain a fair amount of fibre, but when they are milled into flour, such as cornflour, which is used in making instant puddings for example, we do lose this fibre.

There is no particular reason why our dietary fibre should come from bread. If we are eating a varied diet, we will get reasonable amounts of fibre from other foods, particularly from vegetables and from fruit.

Quite a few people these days seem to be sprinkling bran, which is a form of fibre, on to their foods. Having tried it myself, I personally found it to be quite revolting. It seems to me a purely artificial way of going about it and I would much prefer that we adopted normal, sensible, varied diets avoiding too many bland convenience foods, rather than what you might call fads.

If you are worried about roughage, certainly eat wholemeal bread. Many people, I think, prefer it anyway because of its flavour. Eat plenty of leafy vegetables like lettuce, cabbage and cauliflower. They contain plenty of cellulose which the body can't digest, and which is therefore roughage. Fruit contains cellulose too. The general rule is: the more you have to *chew* food, the more roughage it is likely to contain.

Are there nutritional differences between brown breads and white?

Yes, there are; wholemeal bread, as the name implies, contains the whole wheat grain whereas all other types of bread are the result of milling the flour, that is, grinding it up. During the milling process some of the nutrients are lost, more in white bread than in brown. In producing white flour, which we say is of 70 per cent extraction, we lose 30 per cent of the wheat grain. But to allow for that, the nutrients that are lost in milling are added back to white flour when it's made into bread, so in practice we are not really losing anything at all.

Is wheat germ really good for you?

The wheat germ is the seed of the wheat grain, so it's a rich store of different nutrients required for the growing wheat; hence it *is* good for you. Some breads have wheat germ added to them; Hovis is the best-known example. These certainly do contain a greater concentration of nutrients than normal bread; in a normal diet we don't need them.

Should we all bake our own bread?

The answer is no, if we are speaking nutritionally, but for those who have got plenty of time, and who enjoy making bread, then this is a worthwhile recreation. It certainly is an antidote to the growing number of mass-produced products that we tend to have in our diets. But there is nothing special in terms of food value about home-baked bread. It will be just the same as factory bread.

Are sugar substitutes dangerous?

No, they're not bad for us and sugar substitutes, like any new food additive, are subjected to stringent tests. It is true that cyclamate was banned but in fact there is no convincing evidence that if it had not been banned anyone would have suffered, and there's a strong probability, certainly in America, that it will soon be permitted again. In this country the only sugar substitute we can use at the moment is saccharin, which has no food value, and provided that it is taken in moderate amounts, that is normal amounts, there is no danger.

What I mean by normal is this: most of us enjoy an occasional glass of fruit squash. If the sugar in the fruit squash was replaced or partially replaced by saccharin, then we would have a normal average intake of saccharin. If for a week on end we drank nothing but fruit squash, shall we say four or five pints every day, we would then have an abnormal and possibly undesirable intake. But even this sort of level would not necessarily be dangerous because, by law, manufacturers can only add certain amounts and really big safety margins are built in.

Section E Breakfasts and milk

Do we really need the traditional British breakfast? Is this the best way to start the day, and if so, how do the Continentals survive on coffee and a roll?

No, there is no special virtue about the traditional English breakfast. If you happen to enjoy it, by all means eat it, but it has no special merit on its own: milky coffee and a roll and butter can be a perfectly adequate way to start the day in nutritional terms. Continentals enjoy it, I enjoy it, and we seem to live a healthy life.

How important is milk in the diet, both for children and for adults?

It is important because it is the nearest we can get to a perfect food. A perfect food is one which alone would supply all our needs. There is no such thing, but milk approaches it in that it gives a valuable supply of most nutrients, so in any diet it is sensible, though not essential, to include milk both for children and adults. Milk is especially important for children because it provides a good source of calcium, which is required for the formation of bones.

There are some children, of course, who probably do not like, or will not drink, milk. It is possible for them to have an adequate diet without it. Indeed, there are some children who are allergic to cows' milk and alternative diets have to be provided, but I think it is desirable in such cases that the mother should consult a doctor or a dietician to suggest a suitable diet.

There is a possibility of drinking too much milk. It does contain fat; if children were to have too much milk, especially with cream, in the diet, there could be a risk of them becoming obese. But a consumption of around a pint a day is fine.

How do you deal with a child who flatly refuses to eat any breakfast at all?

This sounds to me like a question of rebellion, rather than one of nutrition. If he flatly refuses to eat breakfast, nutritionally speaking he will come to no harm provided that he's willing to eat a normal lunch and other normal meals. There is no magic about eating breakfast as such.

As we saw earlier, the body does appreciate a regular routine and for that reason breakfast is desirable. It has also been shown that breakfast of some sort is desirable in getting the body working, as you might say, in giving us a good start to the day. One point here is that many people feel there is great value in having a hot breakfast 'to beat the cold' but this is completely and absolutely untrue. If we can take a specific example, that well-known Scottish tradition of eating porridge isn't necessarily a good idea, because although it is hot and filling, it contains a lot of water and it's not a sustaining food. You will find that if you start the day on porridge, you are soon going to want a snack mid-day, which rather defeats all good dieting habits. If you have a cold breakfast including some fats your body can get *more* internal energy. The heat of the food is really irrelevant.

Yoghurt seems to have become very popular these days. Is it better than milk?

In a nutritional sense, it's slightly better. They both contain the same nutrients, in fact, but because yoghurt is a more concentrated food than milk, in other words because it contains less water, it does have rather higher levels of nutrients than milk. In particular it contains very approximately half as much protein again as milk. But any magical attribution given to yoghurt is a health food myth. It's made in what might be called a 'natural' way, but this does not affect its food value.

Section F Dieting

How can one diet successfully and not lose energy; that is, can one diet solely on energy-giving foods?

This is an interesting question because really the precise opposite is true. The aim in slimming is to *reduce* our intake of energy-giving foods but not of nutrients that have other functions. We might also add that it is rather unfortunate that we talk about 'diets' when we mean *slimming* diets. We somehow get the feeling there is something special and rather alarming about a diet. In fact the term 'diet' simply means the food that we eat.

But because we want to cut down on the energy-giving foods it does not mean that people on slimming diets should feel less energetic than people who are eating a normal diet. The object of slimming is to lose fat. In other words, obese people have a surplus of fat in the body. The general idea in slimming is to have a greater output of energy than input from food, so that the fat in the body is mobilised to provide us with the energy that we need. Some people are worried that they are going to feel dull and listless if they go on a slimming diet but there is no reason why they should. If you do feel dull and lacking in energy, stop the diet at once.

Is it true that our weight at 21 is where we should stay for the rest of our lives if we are eating properly?

Although in theory bodyweight should not increase with age after 21, in practice with most normal healthy adults there is a slow but gradual increase of weight with age. The point really is that we should eat in such a way that this slight increase in weight doesn't become excessive. For some people there is a reason why at, say 45 years old, they are heavier than they were at 21. Some of us have the happy capacity of burning up our Calories very efficiently. Such individuals find it easy to maintain their weight up to 45; but with others there is a pre-disposition to put on weight; in other words they don't burn Calories up so readily. For them it is probably going to be very difficult to maintain exactly the same weight into middle age.

If we are overweight should we immediately go on a crash diet?

It depends very much on your personality. If you are the sort of person that needs a shock treatment, then a crash diet will probably bring you to your senses. But on the other hand if you're the sort of person who likes the slow haul, the gradual approach, then a crash diet will just be very depressing and it would be far better to go on to a longer-term planned slimming diet.

There is more nonsense talked and there are more fallacies about slimming than perhaps on any other subject. The simple straightforward and short answer is that fat people eat too much and to keep slim you need to eat sensibly. That is, your need is not to go on a diet that will be unenjoyable, but to eat reasonable amounts of food, not excessive amounts. In particular you do have to make sure not to eat too much carbohydrate food. In other words, there is great merit in cutting out foods such as sugar which are pure carbohydrate and provide no other nutrients. But to go on a diet that you hate is to court disaster because you simply won't keep to it.

What is a Calorie-controlled diet, and how important are milk and fat in such a diet?

The name really gives the answer to this question. A Calorie-controlled diet is one in which the number of Calories you consume, or rather the number of Calories produced from the food you consume, is limited. Three nutrients provide us with Calories – those are fats, proteins and carbohydrates – and in a Calorie-controlled diet, all those three nutrients have to be controlled. There are many sets of tables showing the Calorie value of the commonest foods.

Is constipation or diarrhoea a problem when you are dieting?

No, they should be no problem. If the diet is a sensible one, then it will be a *varied diet*, it will provide the nutrients the body requires, and it won't cause those troubles. Looking at the problem the other way round there are certain things that sufferers can do to help overcome them. If you're suffering from constipation, then it would be sensible to make sure that you are getting enough roughage in your diet: make sure that you're eating such things as wholemeal bread, vegetables and fruit. On the other hand, if diarrhoea is the problem then make sure that you are having a bland diet with no very strongly flavoured foods in them. Avoid such things as vinegar and so on. If you do have constipation or diarrhoea for any length of time, don't try and treat it yourself; you must go along to your doctor.

Do we need special diets after illnesses, for example after a heart attack?

Yes, often we do need a special diet, particularly after serious illnesses and particularly after such things as a heart attack, but in such cases, don't take action on your own. Get the advice of a doctor or a dietician. In practical terms after a heart attack it's very likely that a doctor would advise you to cut down on the animal fats in your diet, because there's some evidence, not conclusive, that consumption of animal fats is related to coronary heart disease.

What foods should you eat to put on weight?

The simple answer is that you should eat *more*. Some foods, of course, are more weight enhancing than others: most efficient in this sense are fatty foods because fat is the richest source of Calories. So, for example, eat plenty of fried food, plenty of bread, margarine, fatty meat and so on. I know a few people who have this problem about putting on weight but for most of us I'm afraid the difficulty is exactly the opposite.

Section G   Preparing food at home

Is it dangerous to eat raw vegetables because of chemicals, such as fertilisers and pesticides?

In practical terms, the answer is no. You need not start worrying that you are going to suffer any harm through eating raw vegetables. Perhaps we ought, however, to say that there is a potential danger, which is illustrated by the use of DDT. Back in the 1950s, DDT was widely used as an insecticide and it was discovered that it is such a stable substance that it remains in the soil for many years. The result has been that over the years we have all taken in tiny amounts of DDT with our food. This DDT has become incorporated in our fatty tissues and although no one can prove that this has caused harm, nevertheless it's a cause of concern. Care does need to be exercised in the use of fertilisers and pesticides, and in the case of DDT there has been government action in most countries to ban its use. If you are growing your own vegetables, as many people are, there is a potential danger from the pesticides you may use, but provided you follow the advice given on their use, you will come to no harm.

Which of the vitamins are destroyed in chopping or grating salad vegetables, and which are destroyed in cooking vegetables?

First of all, we need to be clear that the only vitamin that concerns us in both cases is vitamin C. When vegetables are chopped or grated, enzymes are released which cause breakdown of this vitamin. So there is a disadvantage in chopping or grating vegetables finely. Vitamin C is also lost in cooking; the longer a food is cooked, and the higher the temperature that is used, the more vitamin C will be lost. This is the vitamin most easily destroyed, and you've got to take real precautions to preserve it in food.

Are pressure cookers good or bad for keeping nutrients in food?

In fruit and vegetables, the main nutrient that we are likely to lose is vitamin C. Pressure cookers work by using a higher temperature than in boiling, and the higher the temperature the greater the loss of vitamin C. On the other hand, they reduce cooking *time* and this *conserves* vitamin C, so to some extent it's a matter of swings and roundabouts. The net result is rather better retention of vitamin C in pressure cookers than when you boil food in an open pan.

It is not however very significant. In fact, however you cook say, potatoes, it is quite likely that you could lose far more vitamin C by storing the cooked potato, by keeping it hot for, say, half an hour, than you would lose in the cooking process.

Are there some easy practical tips for cooking and serving vegetables to preserve vitamin C?

It's good practice to put the vegetable direct into a minimum of boiling water rather than heat from cold because this kills the enzymes which break down vitamin C. Cook them for as little time as possible and serve and eat them immediately after cooking.

The green colouring in root vegetables, particularly potatoes – to what extent is this poisonous, and could you just cut off the green parts or should you really throw the whole of the potato away?

The green part *is* highly poisonous. It's due to a substance called solanine, which is produced by action of the sun on the potato, but it is quite safe simply to cut out the green part. If by chance small amounts of solanine are left in the potato, then because it is soluble in water, it will be dissolved out when you boil the potatoes. This is purely a potato problem, so you don't have to worry about green patches on swedes or other root vegetables.

Does putting bicarbonate of soda into green vegetables when cooking do anything to them?

If you add small amounts of bicarbonate, it improves the intensity of the green colour, but in case you think that's an advantage, I should add that anything other than a very small amount of bicarbonate produces a mushiness in the texture of the vegetable. It doesn't seem to affect the nutritional value, although there is a suggestion that it could reduce vitamin C levels.

How does tinned baby food compare with food you have prepared yourself?

Really, you can use either, whichever you prefer. Once a baby is over four months old, canned baby food certainly can be convenient and a satisfactory way of feeding them. In very general terms, the canned food will have the same or equivalent nutritional value as the home-prepared food. Perhaps there could be just one or two cautions here. For example, some factory foods (canned baby foods), may tend to be rather sweet. If you use ones which contain sugar, you could be introducing an undesirable habit to the infant. Similarly some of the canned foods do contain additives, large amounts of salt and so on, which you may feel you'd rather your baby did without.

Prior to four months, of course, babies are going to be breast-fed or bottle-fed. Perhaps we could ask the same question here – is it best for mum to feed the baby herself or can the baby do quite well on bottle-feeding preparations based on cows' milk. We have to admit that babies *seem* to thrive, whichever way they are fed, but current thinking is that there is great advantage in the old-fashioned breast-feeding method.

Is it dangerous to warm up cooked meats and vegetables, even if they've been in the fridge or freezer?

Yes, it is certainly highly undesirable and it could even be dangerous to warm up cooked meat. As a matter of good practice, always heat cooked meat right through – cook it to a high temperature and continue cooking until the whole food attains this high temperature. In this way you will kill any germs that might cause harm. The danger in warming up cooked meat is that although it may kill some of the germs, others are more resistant and will not be killed unless high temperatures are used.

As far as vegetables are concerned it certainly is not dangerous to warm them up. Here it is more a matter of deterioration of eating quality.

The fridge and the freezer *do not* kill off the germs that are in your cooked food. You might say they go into hibernation. They are prevented from multiplying, but once the food is taken out of the freezer you must look after it in the same way as you would a fresh food.

Is the best way of roasting joints to do it straight from the freezer, or should they be defrosted first? Will meat lose nutrition by defrosting? Is the fishmonger correct if he says that you don't need to defrost fish before cooking?

It is quite satisfactory to cook the food in its frozen state. This is especially true of food such as fish fingers, cutlets, and so on. If the food is in the form of large pieces, then it is certainly important to cook it thoroughly. If it is being cooked from the frozen state, obviously you have got to supply more heat to cook it than if it started at room temperature, and ideally in such a case you would use a thermometer to check that the food is really cooked right through.

There are some foods where it is not desirable to cook from the frozen state, such as poultry and joints of meat that have been rolled or boned. There is a health hazard from cooking these in the frozen state. This is because of their nature – such foods may contain germs deep within them before they are frozen and these germs may be difficult to kill off if the food is cooked directly from the frozen state. As far as eating meat and fish is concerned, there is certainly no texture advantage in thawing first and in some foods, vegetables for example, you are likely to get a slightly better texture if you cook it straight from the frozen state. Another point is that there are dangers in slow defrosting. If you leave the food lying about for any length of time, the germs which have been inactivated during the freezing will start multiplying again. The secret, whichever way you do it, is to make sure that the food is cooked properly to kill all the germs.

How long can cooked cold meat be kept in the fridge?

There is no single answer to this question and the best we can do is provide some general practical guidelines. First of all, if the cooked food has been prepared in the home, then if it is to be eaten when it is cold, it should not be kept in the fridge for more than 24 hours. On the other hand, if it is to be thoroughly re-heated before it is eaten, you could keep it for a couple of days. If the food was bought in a shop, you could keep it for longer if it contained preservative. For example, sausage meat sold in a packet will have a declaration on the packet if it contains preservatives, and in such a case you could normally keep it for three days.

How can we be sure the food we buy is fresh?

I am afraid the strict answer is that we cannot tell exactly but there are certain points we can look out for. If you know what the fresh food looks like, if you have actually seen it growing, then you know what to look out for. Also, when you see it in the supermarket or wherever you buy it, you can get a general guide to its quality by the way in which it is stored. For example, high quality vegetables and fruit would be stored in the supermarket in a cool cabinet. As far as meats are concerned, it is not easy to give guidelines. The point about good storage conditions obviously still applies, but it is more or less impossible to gauge quality from the colour of the meat. In fact, this can be positively misleading. It is a question of experience and buying food from a reputable retailer.

What effect does freezing, both at home and in the food factory, have on the value of meat and vegetables?

If you mean nutritional value, then it has almost no effect. In terms of nutrients, you lose practically nothing when you freeze a food. When we talk about quality, however, there can be a loss, especially in home freezing. For example, unless vegetables have been properly blanched by pouring hot water over them, enzymes will remain active in the food and will cause deterioration of colour, flavour and possibly texture. If the food has not been blanched, it will not keep in the freezer satisfactorily for more than about six weeks. However, it is important to emphasise the fact that there is no health hazard involved.

Section H   Processed food

How does frozen and canned food compare nutritionally with fresh food?

The quick answer is very well, especially frozen foods, though some will have lost a little vitamin C when they are blanched. But in general, frozen foods and even canned foods may have a higher nutritional value than so-called fresh foods. Canned foods probably will not contain as much vitamin C and thiamine as corresponding fresh foods because the heat processing they have suffered will have caused loss of those two nutrients.

People often assume that nutritional experts would generally recommend people to use fresh foods as opposed to processed foods, but I don't think I would. My opinion is that if you want the highest quality peas for example you are much more likely to get it from frozen peas than from so-called fresh peas. The main reason for this is that when peas are grown for freezing their quality is very carefully controlled while they're being grown, they are only harvested when their quality is at an optimum, and within 90 minutes of harvesting they are frozen. So they've spent a maximum of 90 minutes in transit. If you buy peas in an average shop it is quite likely that they have spent as much as a week since harvesting.

Is it true that tinned food should be taken out of the tin to avoid food poisoning or lead poisoning?

No, I think it's important to appreciate that you certainly will *not* get lead poisoning or food poisoning if you leave food in the can. On the other hand, it is good practice to take the food out of the can. This is mainly because when you open the can you cause some damage around the top of the can, you pierce the lacquer for example and so you can get some attack of the steel of the can from, say, the acid contained in canned fruit. This is not dangerous but taking the fruit out is simply a sensible precaution.

Is it dangerous to eat frozen food past the recommended time?

There is no danger involved at all, but the fact is that very gradually, while food loses eating quality when it is frozen, so that it's undesirable to keep it frozen for too long. In practical terms, regard a year as the maximum time for storing frozen food in a proper freezer where the temperature is maintained at not higher than minus 18°C. In the cold compartment of domestic refrigerators food should be stored for a much shorter length of time because the temperatures are much higher than in a freezer. Here you must be guided by the number of stars on your refrigerator.

Do dehydrated foods (such as soups or dried peas and beans) contain any nutrients at all?

Yes they certainly do. When foods are dehydrated, there is some loss of vitamin C. This is destroyed partly by oxidation and partly by heat; but other nutrients are largely unaffected by the drying process so, for example, proteins and minerals are present just as much in dried food as they were in the original.

Section I   Miscellaneous

Many people today feel tired or lifeless. Aren't there any special foods that they can eat to give them energy and a new zest for life?

Generally speaking, no. Lack of energy and little zest for life are unlikely, in this country, to have a dietary cause. Almost all of us receive enough nutrients to keep us in good health. Iron, for example, will not normally cure tiredness except in special circumstances where, for example, there has been a large loss of blood, and in these cases administration of iron will be necessary. Many foods, particularly so-called 'health foods' with exotic names are promoted as giving people more get-up-and-go. This is complete nonsense. You can buy very expensive preparations with magical properties ascribed to them but these are quite untrue.

Most of us get more energy than we need from food; most of us are trying to cut down on the energy we get from food, and for nearly everybody, being tired or listless certainly isn't the result of an 'unhealthy' diet.

Just a little side issue on this: sometimes we see athletes taking glucose to get 'instant energy'. Glucose certainly does not need to be digested by the body and so the energy in it is rapidly made available. On the other hand, ordinary sugar, sucrose, is rapidly broken down in the body and for all practical purposes there is no advantage in taking glucose rather than sucrose in everyday life. In fact there are really no occasions when the average person needs suddenly to take in sugar for rapid energy because energy is very speedily made available from resources already within the body.

Are there any specific foods that you can eat to make you healthier and fitter?

Everyday food does keep you healthy and fit. It's true that there are some preparations on the market which manage to convey the impression that if only you will eat them, you will become fitter. This is usually attributed to vitamins and mineral elements that they contain. On the whole, if you are eating a normal, varied diet, then use of these preparations is a complete and utter waste of money.

Are any foods good for the nerves? Is depression caused by what we eat or what we don't eat?

Only if the nervous condition is due to some particular lack in the diet, notably lack of vitamins. Because most people in this country do have a satisfactory diet, they certainly should *not* immediately blame any 'nerves' or depression that they may have on the diet. If they are in doubt, then they should consult a doctor. There are no specific foods which are good for 'nerves', or for depression.

Can a mother pass on her eating habits to her baby during pregnancy, when a baby's in the womb?

No, she can't, but on the other hand it is clear that the mother's eating habits during pregnancy do affect the well-being and the growth of the unborn baby. She can get advice on the best diet at her ante-natal clinic. As soon as the baby is born, then the mother can instil good or bad eating habits into her baby.

Why don't schools teach more about nutrition?

I think schools would be rather upset by that question. They spend a fair amount of energy in trying to teach nutrition. In recent years we've seen that this subject has become accepted not only for girls but also for boys. But basically, there is only a certain amount that *can* be taught about nutrition in a school: information on its own is not enough. When we are talking about nutrition, we are talking about the food that we eat, we are talking about something that is practical. The only way of learning nutrition is to carry it out in practice, so that if children are going to learn more, the example that they see and follow in the home is just as important as the teaching that they get at school.

Acknowledgements

Acknowledgement is due to the following for permission to reproduce photographs:
DAVID ATTENBOROUGH aborigines, page 46; BARNABY'S PICTURE LIBRARY Scotsman (A. W. Besley), page 11; BIRDS EYE FOODS LTD. freezing peas, page 74; BRITISH MUSEUM banquet, page 16; BRITISH MUSEUM (NATURAL HISTORY) hunting, pages 8–9, farming, page 10; BRITISH OXYGEN CO. LTD. freezer plant, page 117; CAMERA PRESS spaghetti (J. P. Chatelin), page 40, child with marasmus (Bo-Erik Gyberg), page 113, New Guinea man (Richard Harrington), page 116; C.O.I. shepherd, page 12; CRODA FOOD INGREDIENTS multi-plate freezer, pages 72–73; H. J. HEINZ CO. LTD. canning plant, page 66; LONDON SCHOOL OF HYGIENE & TROPICAL MEDICINE child with kwashiorkor, page 113; MANSELL COLLECTION cookery book illustration, page 43; MUSÉE DE LOUVRE, PARIS Rembrandt's "Bathsheba", page 82; NATIONAL MAGAZINE CO. LTD. meat pie and vegetables, page 41, all photographs page 62; DR. E. G. J. OLSEN, NATIONAL HEART HOSPITAL healthy and diseased arteries, pages 86 and 87; RADIO TIMES HULTON PICTURE LIBRARY kitchen, page 15, baking, pages 18–19, banquets, pages 44 and 45, jam-making, pages 64–65, cartoon, page 80, sugar milling, pages 90–91 and 93; RHM RESEARCH LTD. starch, pages 35 and 36; SYNDICATION INTERNATIONAL curry, page 41; UNITED NATIONS goitre, page 49; WEST INDIA COMMITTEE LIBRARY windmill, page 92.

Acknowledgement is also due to the following:
DAVIS-POYNTER LTD for extract from *The Western Way of Death* by Malcolm Carruthers; GERALD DUCKWORTH & CO. LTD. for extract from 'On Food' by Hilaire Belloc from *Cautionary Tales*; FABER & FABER LTD. for extract from *Food – Facts & Fallacies* by Allan Cameron; THE LITERARY TRUSTEES OF WALTER DE LA MARE, AND THE SOCIETY OF AUTHORS AS THEIR REPRESENTATIVE for extract from 'Miss T'. by Walter de la Mare; MACGIBBON & KEE for extract from *The New Apocrypha: A Guide to Strange Sciences and Occult Beliefs* by John Sladek; MERLIN PRESS LTD. for extract from *Can Britain Feed Itself?* by Kenneth Mellanby; JOHN MURRAY (PUBLISHERS) LTD. for extract from *Food & Society* by Magnus Pyke.

Food in History by Reay Tannahill (Paladin paperback).

Cover illustration by Mick Brownfield. Drawings in the text are by Ray Burrows and Corrine Clarke, the cartoons are by David Mostyn.